KNOCKING MYSELF UP

knocking myself up

A MEMOIR OF MY (IN)FERTILITY

---

michelle tea

DEYST.

An Imprint of WILLIAM MORROW

DEYST.

KNOCKING MYSELF UP. Copyright © 2022 by Michelle Tea. All rights reserved. Printed in the United States of America. No part of this book may be used or reproduced in any manner whatsoever without written permission except in the case of brief quotations embodied in critical articles and reviews. For information, address HarperCollins Publishers, 195 Broadway, New York, NY 10007.

HarperCollins books may be purchased for educational, business, or sales promotional use. For information, please email the Special Markets Department at SPsales@harpercollins.com.

A hardcover edition of this book was published in 2022 by Dey Street, an imprint of William Morrow.

FIRST DEY STREET PAPERBACK EDITION PUBLISHED 2023.

Designed by Angela Boutin

Library of Congress Cataloging-in-Publication Data

Names: Tea, Michelle, author.
Title: Knocking myself up : a memoir of my (in)fertility / Michelle Tea.
Description: First edition. | New York, NY : Dey St., an imprint of William Morrow, [2022]
Identifiers: LCCN 2022018377 (print) | LCCN 2022018378 (ebook) | ISBN 9780063210622 (hardcover) | ISBN 9780063210639 (paperback) | ISBN 9780063210806 (ebook) | ISBN 9780063210653 | ISBN 9780063210660
Subjects: LCSH: Tea, Michelle. | Women authors, American—21st century—Biography. | Lesbian authors—United States—Biography. | Fertility clinics—United States. | Fertilization in vitro, Human—United States.
Classification: LCC PS3570.E15 Z46 2022 (print) | LCC PS3570.E15 (ebook) | DDC 813/.54 [B]—dc23/eng/20220520
LC record available at https://lccn.loc.gov/2022018377
LC ebook record available at https://lccn.loc.gov/2022018378

ISBN 978-0-06-321063-9

23 24 25 26 27 LBC 5 4 3 2 1

For Tara Jepsen

contents

2013

ONE OUT OF FOUR; OR, DISAPPOINTMENT

2014

INVASION OF THE BODY SNATCHER; OR, JOY

2021

INTRODUCTION

Hello. This is your narrator, Michelle Tea. I'm about to bring you into my inner world, during a period of time when that space was as wild, messy, hopeful, dizzy, tragic, terrifying, and openhearted as any era I've ever lived. The process of deciding to have a baby and then going through with it is a rollicking ride regardless of who you are and what your situation might be. You're setting out to conjure a life, and in the process, deeply unsettle your own. The you that you know yourself to be is about to be forever changed, not just by the introduction of a whole new person into the world, but by the decision itself, the places—literal and figurative—it takes you, the way it forces you to think differently about who you are and how you live. Every birth story is this; not just the dramatic climax of a last push and a first breath, but the story of a choice made, a dare accepted, a journey undertaken. The whole story of a birth begins with that decision to say *yes*, and the roller coaster that loop-de-loops you to the delivery table or at-home birthing pool or what have you—there is so much in it.

All of life, every hope and fear, joy and sadness, the understanding of yourself as a mammal, an embodied animal, is in that story.

Whether you've had kids or want to someday or thank your lucky stars on the regs that you are child-free and therefore FREE; whether you're trapped in ambivalence about this big question, if you ended a pregnancy, are seeking to adopt, to foster, or plan to stick with cats; whether your body can nurture this kind of life or not, I hope you find in my story what we all look for in a book: a gaze into someone else's life that removes us, temporarily, from our own, that leaves us with new perspectives. I hope you laugh when it's funny and feel a smidge of my pain when it's not. For those of you who are contemplating this big life question, how cool if my own experience can help you weigh the pros and cons or, if appropriate, inspire you to leap into the unknown? For those considering such a quandary who, like me, felt on the outside of traditional mom culture—because you're queer or broke, unpartnered or uninsured, because you don't look like our culture's stereotype of the white, trim, middle-class, sexless mother—I really hope you find in my voice a kindred spirit.

When I set out to try to knock myself up, I had pledged to not be precious about it. I would resist what the culture expects of people choosing to reproduce; I would resist the idea that this was the most important, most sacred thing I could ever do. At forty, I'd already done a lot, and many of those things were real accomplishments as important as breeding. I wanted to keep potential motherhood in its proper place—life-changing and magical, sure, but also incredibly common, one identity among many intersecting identities, one peak in a mountain range. Yes, the stakes become higher, but a sense of irreverence, deep (sometimes macabre) humor, a challenging eye, a gossipy tone—these are things I wanted to reflect in this journey, to help humanize it, wrench it away from the contemporary culture of precious mommyhood, into something more relatable and accessible.

I truly wasn't sure I wanted a kid when I jumped off this cliff; I said *yes* more as a way to break out of what felt like a stultifying ambivalence, a dare to the Universe to solve the issue for me—give me a baby or don't—so I could move past a question that weighed more heavily with each passing year. Somewhere in the multiverse is a me who didn't get pregnant, who instead moved to Paris and is currently bringing coffee and croissants to her throuple *lovers* lounging in their big bed in a tiny room in a Pigalle walk-up. Somewhere else is a me who adopted; somewhere else is a me who got knocked up naturally in my heterosexual youth—that me is a grandmother now. Our lives swirl with possibilities always, directions taken and refused. I set forth on this one and found turning back from it to be impossible. In this iteration of the multiverse, I'm Mom, the kind of mom who got here through an odd yet common, queer, and privileged path. I hope you enjoy the adventure.

2011

THE BIOLOGICAL
CLOCK; OR, OPTIMISM

1.

A COLD SUMMER NIGHT
IN SAN FRANCISCO

When I started telling the people around me that I was going to get myself pregnant, they reacted in a variety of ways, and not always as expected. My two best friends, with whom I have a very code*friend*ent relationship, were skeptical. "You can't just go and put the baby in the other room when you want to have sex," Tali said wryly, an apparent comment on my amorous lifestyle. Tali and I have been friends since the nineties, when we were both drunken poets slurring into the mic at open-mic events. Now that we were older, and sober, Tali's approach to life had become more grounded and cautious, and she was unafraid to offer her strong opinions, peppered as they were with a dark and honest humor.

I was uncertain how to respond to my dear friend's read—of *course* I understood that the baby would have to come before my libido, but, really, why couldn't I tuck the baby in the other room when I wanted to have sex? That sounded reasonable. Tali tried another angle: "You like to take off and go to Paris." I was becoming a bit enchanted with my life as seen through my friend's eyes. Who was this jet-setting tart? But I hadn't been to Paris in years, and anyway, wouldn't I *want* to take my little bohemian baby traveling abroad? Wouldn't I want to teach them French by immersion in the cafés of the Bastille? In fact, maybe I would want to actually *give birth* in Paris, gifting my *bébé* with dual citizenship in an elegant, socialist country and treating myself to a free, socialist hospital birth! Tali saw that her warnings were having the opposite effect and sighed in resignation, offering one more deterrent: "But you *love* your life."

This made me pause: *I do love my life,* I thought to myself. I lived by myself in a spacious San Francisco apartment I could miraculously afford with the income I patched together running a literary nonprofit, writing books and essays, and reading tarot cards. My apartment building was old and gray, but in a dignified way, like Iris Apfel. The staircase had a polished wood banister, and the lobby was lined with mirrors, so you could get your Last Lewks in before you pushed open the heavy glass door and went out onto the wind tunnel that is Page Street.

Landing there seemed like a miracle in and of itself; not least because my inbred money scarcity almost pushed me to turn my back on it. The fact that the rent was seriously under market value—this, during the legendary San Francisco era of the Tech Bro!—did not even register to me. All I saw was that it was more money than I'd ever spent on housing, and I balked, fear of having to come up with more money per month setting my stomach churning. Thankfully, some friends who, while they may be similarly blinded by their own survival fears, can at least see it plain and clear when manifesting in another. "That entire apartment literally costs *two hundred dollars more* a month than what you're paying to live in a converted living room in a flat with twentysomethings who keep mistaking their cocaine panic for heart attacks and calling the fire department," Tali lectured sternly. "You should move."

San Francisco is a city of neighborhoods, but this latest spot I found myself in, my charmed apartment, seemed to be in a liminal space. I'd lived in a few different San Francisco neighborhoods—mostly the Mission, which I watched go from a neighborhood of Latinx families, Salvadoran restaurants, street hookers, and dykes to a neighborhood of white tech workers, pastry shops selling deconstructed confections, electric scooters, and yoga moms. For years I lived in North Beach, worried the throngs of tourists would drive me mad, but I was ultimately delighted to be residing in a spot that so many people, from all around the world, wanted to visit. The air smelled like rosemary focaccia, and my local bookstore was City Lights, where the elderly Lawrence Ferlinghetti (RIP) was often in residence, being interviewed by European film crews. I'd also lived in Bernal Heights, both at the foggy top of the hill, where condensation would drift beneath the back door and fill the kitchen with clouds, and at the bottom, where the jagged singsong of drunkards doing karaoke at Nap's provided a quirky soundtrack to my life. My new neighborhood was a no-man's-land that wasn't quite the grungy Lower Haight and wasn't quite Hayes Valley. It was a lovely spot that allowed me to walk most anywhere, or hop on a lumbering orange bus if it was rainy or I was lazy.

After decades cohabiting with various roommates, I relished the luxury of my own apartment. Nobody left passive-aggressive notes for me if I didn't clean up my mess swiftly enough. No having to nag people for their portion of the electric bill. No facing another human in the kitchen before I'd had my first cup of coffee. Life was pretty blissful, and when I thought about my humble beginnings, across the country in a run-down New England town, my life felt like a freaking fairy tale. Which was exactly why I wanted to bring a little creature into it! From where I stood, deep into my fortieth year on earth, my remaining eggs hobbling down my fallopian tubes each month, tennis balls wedged onto their walkers, it seemed like having a kid was the only adventure I *hadn't* undertaken.

My friend Mel's face crumpled in despair when I told them. "Your work!" they moaned, mourning all the books I would not write. They told me all about the depressing life of their girlfriend's sister, a single mother. Everyone, it seemed, had stories of miserable single mothers and they all wanted to share them with me.

And yet all the moms I knew were totally psyched and encouraging of my steps toward Babyville. My AA sponsor, deeply in love with her adopted son, urged me on, suggesting I have an affair while traveling. In their thirties, while selling weed, my friend Belle accidentally got knocked up by their bipolar boyfriend and kept the baby; now they have a second kid and live an inspiring life in Hollywood working on television projects (sans bipolar boyfriend). They racked their brain for sperm donors, briefly offering up their husband, but then realized they'd be upset if my baby wound up better than theirs. Esther, another writer who kept her accidental pregnancy, also thought it was a great idea. We remembered sitting backstage with Exene Cervenka at a poetry reading, how she urged us to have a kid someday. "It makes you more psychic," she promised, a nice perk.

My sister Madeline, who not only had a three-year-old daughter but who knows me better than anyone—my strengths and weaknesses, how I am both diligent and a space cadet—began teaching me how to track my ovulation cycle. My mother, a lovable nervous wreck who is often frightened of my life choices (sex work, walking through the East Village alone past midnight, attending Mayan sweat lodges in the Mexican jungle), surprised me by offering advice on turkey basters. How did she know about this classic, lesbian method of insemination? Floating on their encouragement, it seemed that I was—with a lingering hint of trepidation—really pursuing this! With my mom on board, how could even my most reticent friends not come around? Tali, who supports her writing habit by working in a co-op grocery store, relented: "Well, I can get you twenty percent off your prenatal vitamins. And tell your mom we have really high-quality glass turkey basters."

Although my friends' anti-baby fears gave me the opportunity to try out my pro-baby arguments, the truth was, the dare to depart in this wild new direction existed inside my body alongside self-doubt, the economic scarcity issues that were my birthright, and basic terror of the unknown. My inner *Yes* and *No* merged into a gray fog of ambivalence. I wanted to know, with a bright, clear one hundred percent assurance that *Yes,* a child was totally my destiny and would make my life complete, or *No,* I was simply not cut out for motherhood, what with my head for art and my bod for sin and my income that fluctuated like a PMS mood swing.

Throughout my twenties, I thought of pregnancy the same way I thought of any STD, but with a dose of the movie *Alien.* Something foreign gestates inside you, siphoning your nutrients, changing your behaviors (as many parasites do), before finally clawing its way out, leaving you maimed and possibly even dead. Many acquaintances were disturbed by this understanding of babies as invasive monsters and not, you know, *cute.*

Then, at twenty-seven, I read Ariel Gore's book *The Hip Mama Survival Guide* and suddenly pregnancy seemed sort of cool, like some sort of wild art project. Ariel's book was the first thing I had ever read that gave *me*—poor, queer, weird—permission to bring a kid into the world. I don't know if the book triggered something biological or if it was right time, right place, but suddenly babies didn't seem like the grotesque hobgoblins I'd feared them to be. In fact, I began craving the feeling of being pregnant. *What is this?* I marveled. How could my body crave something it had never known? This new sensation surged briefly into an obsession before it receded, leaving me different. The thought of having a kid was no longer repulsive.

For the next decade, I wobbled back and forth, wondering if a child was something I wanted. It was frustrating not to know. I had a long-term relationship with someone who absolutely did *not* want a baby, who got worked into a frenzy if the topic was introduced even speculatively, causing me to shelve it. Later, I dated people who *did* want children, but they tended to suffer from borderline personality disorder or some Not Otherwise Specified psychological malaise. It seemed that if I had a healthy partner who wanted a baby, then maybe *I* would want a baby, too. I began to lament the impossibility of getting *accidentally* knocked up. When I was younger, I was relieved that the people I dated—women, trans men, and gender nonconforming people assigned female at birth—could not get me pregnant. What a great thing not to have to worry about. Now I was regretful that I couldn't allow a broken condom to make the decision for me.

All of this brings me to a cold summer night in San Francisco, when I sat at my vintage kitchen table, a cheery, buttercup-yellow Formica, my laptop displaying what appeared to be a legit source detailing how tragic my forty-year-old eggs were. Horrifyingly, I learned, your eggs are best during the fragile era of your late teens/ early twenties. By the time you're forty, you are 46 percent likely not to get pregnant; in just five years that rises to 58 percent. If I wanted a baby, I would have to do it right then. Like, right that very second. But I wasn't in a real relationship! I had allowed a somewhat recent heartbreak to slingshot me into a rebound with a person who was likewise rebounding from their own heartbreak. This fake relationship provided us both with an excellent diversion from the fact that we were sort of still in love with our respective exes. We wrote poetry together, attended the county fair, arrived at avant-garde art events arm in arm, and spent our workdays contributing to an excitingly perverse G-Chat thread set in the broom closet of a Catholic high school, featuring a janitor and *moi*. We even spoke wistfully about running away to New York City to start an art gallery, or to Amsterdam to be hookers. But despite the idyllic picture I'm painting, our connection was marred by the simple fact that our hearts were elsewhere.

There, at my kitchen table in the June of my fortieth year, the mandate seemed clear: get out of my fake relationship, find someone hot and not insane who wanted to have a baby ASAP, and get to bonding on the double so that we'd be ready to take this life-changing step together by the end of the year. And so, I began to cry. But the crying, I shortly realized, was good! The crying was *very* good! I was finally having a definite feeling about having a kid! Look how inconsolable I got when it seemed I couldn't have one! I *did* want one! I clicked shut my computer, flipped a tarot card, and regarded the High Priestess and all her introspective self-knowing, her solitary femme power and overall positive vibes. I broke up with my fake date. And I decided to have a baby.

2.

DR. MOODY BUTCH

The websites that had made me cry about the shabby state of my eggs also urged me to talk to an actual doctor. And so I went to my clinic, a sliding-scale joint for the uninsured that shares a floor with an AA clubhouse. You never know what you're going to get at the clinic. On this particular day, I was met with the surprise of a brand-new doctor. Apparently, my old MD, whom I adored, required greater job security than the clinic—with its righteous mission statement and rocky funding sources—could provide. My new doc, a moody butch with gelled hair, looked at me blankly when I told her I wanted to have a baby.

"And is there a problem?"

"No," I said. "Just, um, all the websites said I should talk to a doctor, because I'm forty."

"You still getting your period?"

"Yes," I said.

"Do you have a partner?"

"No, I'm just going to, you know, ask some fags to give me

sperm." I chuckled and smiled, trying to loosen her up with a homosexual in-joke. Nothing.

"Also, I take Celexa," I told Dr. Moody Butch. "Will I have to go off my meds?"

"I don't think so," she said. "There may be some serotonin withdrawal in the infant, but you should be able to stay on them."

Serotonin withdrawal! That sounded like a horrible way to enter the planet! As a now-clean drug addict who once whiled away the day waiting for my crystal meth–kidnapped serotonin to return, I could think of nothing worse. No serotonin equals feeling like you want to die. I couldn't imagine how fucked a person's brain chemistry would be, starting their life like that. But then, starting life with a wackadoodle, off-her-meds mama was no doubt just as stressful.

I left the clinic with a purse full of multivitamins called Go Folic!, named for the local public health initiative, which produced them for moms-to-be. I felt like there were a million things I should have asked the doctor, and there were. For instance, my friend Monica, whose partner had their kid via natural birth when she was forty-three years old, scolded me for not inquiring about an FSH test.

"What's an FSH test?" I asked her.

"A follicle-stimulating hormone test," explained Monica. "If your eggs are elderly and have a hard time making it down the tubes, your body will produce this hormone to give it a kick down the chute. Elevated FSH means your eggs are *not* awesome and you'll have a hard time getting pregnant." It seemed essential. I called the clinic back to request one.

"Dr. Moody Butch said you don't need one," the receptionist told me.

"But I want one," I pushed.

"She said try for six months and then come back if you're not pregnant."

This made me want to cry. I wasn't sure how I would get pregnant, but I knew it would not be easy. It would require cajoling reticent gay boys into handing over some of their magic mucus, if not purchasing it outright for thousands of dollars from a sperm bank. Six months of futile sperm bank visits was not an option, economically.

"I need to know if I can get pregnant before I begin trying," I insisted.

"I'm sorry, that's not how we do it," she maintained.

Instead of an FSH test, I went to Walgreens and appraised a shelf I had never looked twice at: the back wall stacked with pregnancy tests, ovulation tests, fertility tests, newfangled clit ticklers, condoms, lube, and scented pussy wipes. That day, I was shopping for my first of many—*many*—pee sticks, this one a stick of treated paper designed to detect the presence of the dreaded follicle-stimulating hormone in my urine.

On the third day of my period, a period that seems to get alarmingly weirder every month—is this it? Is this *the last egg?*—I peed on a stick and waited to see what would happen. A single, hot pink line appeared in the little window. Was that good or bad? I couldn't remember! I was keyed up and spazzy. Wait—it was good. No FSH. My eggs were still sashaying down the tubes unassisted. In two more days it would be day five of my period, and I could purchase a box of ovulation pee sticks and begin tracking when I was fertile. I was really on my way now, down the single-use-plastic-pee-stick-strewn path trod by so many women before me.

3.

YOU HAD ME AT WARM BOWL

There are a few methods for a baby-hungry woman to obtain sperm. My preferred choice was bumming sperm off one of the hot gay boys I was acquainted—but not *too* well acquainted—with. I wasn't looking for a co-parent. I just wanted a nice, casual transfer of fluids and a willingness to meet the kid when they turn fourteen and start asking who their dad is. Or I could just have sex with some guy and get myself knocked up. Being mostly gay, I'd barely had a one-night stand with a strange man, but having watched many movies, it seemed like all I'd have to do was sit alone in a bar, perhaps in the flattering glow of a wall sconce, wearing a body-con dress, and a man would come to me.

Bernadine told me about a lesbian who had put an ad on Craigslist and found a guy to fuck her every month until she got pregnant, which she did. She never even learned the guy's name, and he never learned hers. Bernadine was an all-business Capricorn, and I could feel her pleasure at finding me a way to cut corners. I did feel relief knowing that, if all else failed, I could get pregnant on Craigslist!

But Craigslist was second choice, after soliciting sperm from a friend but before going to a sperm bank, which seemed too expensive—a single batch of sperm ran about $1,500—and sort of clinical. "You've spent that much on a purse," my sister scolded me. Which is true. But I had both a posh teaching job and a posh book advance when I bought that purse, neither of which I had now. *And* I don't drive, so have no car payments, and am not even bothering to save to buy a home someday, it's so far from my reality, so why not blow a magical windfall on a fancy purse? Just because I did it once doesn't make it a *lifestyle*. It is also worth mentioning that I wouldn't have to go back to Barneys every month and buy yet *another* Balenciaga bag when the previous bag failed to get me pregnant. Then, there is the fact that I *hate* paying for things I can get for free. Not to mention my suspicion toward these sperm-donating guys? Who even were they? My evil lesbian ex-girlfriend had almost donated her eggs and had lied through her teeth about everything. Some dudes desperate to jerk off for one hundred dollars would no doubt be lying about their alcoholic moms or their bipolar dads or call themselves creative, when arranging a plate of nachos for their Super Bowl party was as creative as it got. It was also harder to get pregnant from sperm bank sperm, the jizz having been frozen and manhandled and whatnot. I wasn't going down that money pit unless I had to, and with so much free sperm walking around, it didn't seem like I did.

I started sending really awkward emails to fags. Moving relationships that existed mainly at bars and performance spaces from a casual "Hey, girl, what's up," to inquiring about something as intimate as the sharing of bodily fluids and the specter of behind-the-scenes parenthood—via *email*—was weird, but I was determined. I asked an incredibly beautiful performance artist—last seen shoving a lit candle up his ass—via Facebook, and asked many more people in person, causing them to shift with discomfort and make self-deprecating jokes about their genes. Incidentally, many friends expressed concern about my future baby getting "good genes." Good genes include tallness, a lack of alcoholism, and no mental illness. Fair enough, but as a short alcoholic on Celexa, I presumed my offspring would likely be shrimpy and anxious, with a predisposition for problem drinking; it's just something I'd have to watch for as a parent. Also, if nearly everything is genetic—which I believe may be so—perhaps a capacity for sobriety could also be passed along. With this in mind, I began actively seeking donors who were sober alcoholics, but not considering anyone who was presently a hot mess.

ALL AROUND ME ARE WOMEN WITH LITTLE BABIES. OR GOOFY TODDLERS. OR giant alien pregnancy bellies. As I have a croissant in a café, a woman wheels her infant past and I am gripped with the desire to grab her and ask, *Where did you get your sperm?* Because I am a narcissist or something, I forget that most mothers did not have to scrounge around for a scarce squirt of sperm. *I bet you just forgot to put a condom on, didn't you?* I think as I glower privately at a woman passing by, a baby bouncing in its Björn upon her giant, milked-up cleavage. Then I sigh mournfully into my coffee and get on with my day.

I have a Skype with my genius ex-boyfriend Lindsey, who is off in Canada studying how to become a bigger genius in some super-exclusive program full of crazy genius nerds. "Quentin is dying to give his sperm away," he suggests. Quentin is one of Lindsey's best friends, a baby drag queen who performs under the name Miss Super Extra Deluxe Pandemonium. She wears a lot of makeup and bright eighties shoulder pads, and her drag queen hair is my actual ideal hair—a sort of curly, frizzy, halo-y, big, long Jewfro. Miss Super Extra Deluxe Pandemonium is a "chosen person" who hosts drag bat mitzvahs. In his non-drag life, Quentin is an exceptionally adorable gay boy who works for nonprofits and wears fun outfits like sweater vests and bow ties, or brightly colored tank tops and daisy dukes. He was involved in cool political campaigns and had recently asked if I would be part of a date auction to benefit a mayoral candidate too good to actually win. For twenty years I had managed to avoid being date-auctioned, a scenario I thought embarrassing, a bit pompous, and not really the best moneymaker. But I would do anything for Quentin, so I said yes, and a book-shopping date with me was now available for purchase.

I sent Quentin an email with the subject line *A Krazy Kwestion*. I imagined circus music and a little dog hula-hooping. His response was swift.

Hey Michelle!
Wow, I'm totally honored! And I think I'd be up for it, but would like to think a bit more about it before giving you a final yes. I will say that I once tried to donate to the sperm bank in Berkeley, but I was too short (full disclosure: I am 5'6"!).

Hi Quentin!
Oh my god, I can't believe you got turned down for SHORTNESS! That is GENDER OPPRESSION! Short people are the cutest! I don't care about that. With my genetics, I think I can expect a short alcoholic. Bring it!

I went on to explain to Quentin that he would basically pleasure himself somewhere in my house, deposit his man-magic in a warm bowl, and that one of my dear friends would bring it to where I lay, with my feet in the air, awaiting impregnation.

You had me at warm bowl, Quentin replied. Oh my god oh my god oh my god! I had my donor! A twentysomething, adorable, attractive, artistic, intelligent, politically conscious, super funny *gay boy!* Who is also Jewish! I don't know *why* Jewish should be a bonus, actually, but it just felt special. Everyone knows Jewish people are special. Quentin's willingness to say yes to this baby caper was hugely validating: something about my zany spirit must also be maternal if this charming, smart young man was willing to contribute his sperm to the cause. I felt frozen with both excitement and fear. I'd put something into motion, and it was moving.

4.

THEN I MET ORSON

In the midst of this, I began to date someone. I did not have any type of plan to date anyone, ever again. My recent track record of crashed-and-burned miniature "relationships" had led me to some conclusions. Something inside me, some sex-crazed, beastly aspect of my astrology—say, my Sagittarius stellium—or perhaps something compulsive and pleasure-seeking connected to my alcoholism made me capable of having tragically great sex with really awful people, then mistaking the postcoital onslaught of chemicals for *true love*. After going around this crazy carousel a dozen or so times, I was dizzy and sickened by my own repetitive delusions, and I wanted *off*. I would from here on out sink all my love energy into my writing and my future offspring. No more boys, or boy-girls, or girl-boys, or any sexy gender combinations for me.

Beneath the extreme lack of faith I had in my ability to make sound romantic choices lurked a darker, sadder "conclusion": that love, romantic love, *didn't actually exist,* that it was but an amalgamation of codependence and sexual urge, festooned with delusions fostered by a culture hell-bent on shoving idealized notions of couplehood down our throats. I don't know why the culture should care so much about us all being coupled up, but it did. Maybe because love was a distraction that kept us from overthrowing capitalism? To prop up heterosexist "family values"? Whatever the reason, everyone was brainwashed, but not me, not anymore.

Then I met Orson.

It happened at the date auction, where they had come to go dancing with their ex-girlfriend, who was also their bestie. Orson looks like the lost Curtis brother from *The Outsiders,* the one who just could not handle the *chaos* of that household and went off and got himself an apartment and a little Maltese Terrier mutt and lived a tidy and serene life away from the greaser-soc gang violence. Orson was very polite and asked me a spate of sort of wholesome questions that were very charming, like where I grew up and what I'd had for breakfast that day, and then they asked me out via text. Days later they came and picked me up at my door like a gentleman and hailed a gentlemanly cab and took us to this really lovely seafood restaurant and then walked me home and then we made out and *guess what?* It made me super dizzy! Being a new woman, I was determined to *go slow,* something I really didn't know how to do, but I figured not having sex on the first date was probably a good start. I couldn't just date any old fool if I had a baby coming. Not only did they have to be relationship material, they also sort of had to be *dad material.*

I kept waiting for Orson to unzip their face. They seemed too good to be true. They had a good job and they liked their mom. They kept buying me dinner. They laughed at my jokes. They seemed *happy.* Okay, I thought, as we shared a pizza, *this is the date where they're going to get weird, and I'll get uncomfortable, and thus will begin the long, sad, drawn-out process of me pretending they didn't make me uncomfortable, ignoring that rising panic that begins when I know someone is unzipping their face but I'm pretending they're not because I'm just "giving them a chance."* As Orson continued to not unzip their face, at the close of our second date—dinner at a fancy pizza place, where we talked our heads off about our families and childhoods and rotten exes—I was hit with a pang of guilt that, despite all I'd shared, I still hadn't told them I was about to maybe probably hopefully get pregnant.

5.

THE THIRD DATE

There is only one candidate for the Bearer of the Warm Bowl, that person who shall ferry the Pyrex of drag queen sperm from my kitchen to my bedroom: my bestie, Rhonda. Rhonda is like a non-stoner, female Jeff Spicoli who is a landscaper by day and a performance artist/stand-up comic by night. In between day and night, she is a late-in-life lady skateboarder who takes feral tweenaged boys of all backgrounds under her wing, bringing them to the skate park and buying them helmets when their moms are too busy spending their cash on personalized license plates for their Beamers. Sometimes Rhonda has her platinum hair all sexy and discoed out and she's wearing cute, voluminous frocks, and other times she is in flip-flops and cutoffs singing Van Halen in the karaoke bar attached to the bowling alley in Daly City.

Rhonda is the perfect Bearer of the Warm Bowl for many reasons. We have been friends since 1995 and have seen each other through all sorts of embarrassing hairdos (pink crew cuts, green extensions) and even more embarrassing romantic choices. A Scorpio, she is a complex mixture of townie hard-ass and teary tenderheart, and she does not shy away from intense situations. She is also *dying* for me to have a baby, which is crucial. Overall, Rhonda is not grossed out by life, and when I ask her if she'll carry the bowl—which, let's be real, does not entail *only* transporting a warm bowl of splooge but also sucking it up into a syringe of sorts and then assisting with the *insertion* of the syringe and pushing the plunger—well, Rhonda cries a bit. So I know I've selected the right person. Counting fourteen days from the start of my period (I was told by a mother of two that I'll ovulate between fourteen and seventeen days), I draw a big red star in my Moleskine planner and invite Quentin and Rhonda over for our first insemination party, two weeks hence.

With a date on the calendar, I am sweating it hard with Orson. I am someone who tends to lay all my cards on the table in the first fifteen minutes of meeting someone. I overshare. I'm TMI, 24–7. Add to this chatty impulse a sort of warped codependency that makes me feel like I'm being totally dishonest if I don't reveal everything about myself to someone I like the minute I start liking them, and I am in a state. Luckily, I surround myself with stauncher females; stoic, hardened bitches who know how to play a courtship. I begin with Bernadine. I have a bit of learned helplessness with Bernadine. She always has the answers to everything, so often, instead of figuring things out for myself, I just ask her.

Bernadine, I text, *on what date with Orson do I tell them I'm going to get pregnant?*

If you want to tell them anything—which you're not required to do here—just be honest about your plans to get knocked up while you're still fertile. I think date number three, she responds. My heart flops around in my chest. Date number three is that night!

I decide I need a chorus of opinions and also consult Rhonda. *Does it feel like the connection is deepening?* she asks. Totally! Because there is this sort of gorgeous *goodness* that spills from handsome Orson's very aura, I am feeling very connected to them! We stare into each other's eyes for so long, if any of my friends saw us they would laugh and blow spitballs into my hair and I would not even *notice,* so transfixed by Orson am I! Orson uses the word *fresh.* Like, when I tease them flirtatiously, they blush and say, "Are you being fresh?" Who *says* that? *Olde tyme-y* people like Orson, who dress as Mr. Rogers for Halloween and play obscure soul music while perfecting their side parts in the bathroom mirror. Orson and I have both been burned by past loves in almost *the exact same way!* It's uncanny. Yes, the connection is deepening, but I feel it hit a wall, because I am keeping this very big secret. I'm holding them a bit at arm's length, because chances are they'll bolt, and who could blame them? What thirty-two-year-old queer wants to learn that the lady they're hooking up with is about to morph into a forty-year-old *mom?*

Three dates in, Rhonda eventually says, and again I'm shook. I ask my friend Naz, one of the most opinionated people I know. She is also the first butch person I have asked, and I wonder if her opinion will differ from the finger-snapping *you don't owe no one nothing* attitude of my femme-centric friends.

OMG first date definitely!!! Naz screams at me via text. *Um, too late for that*, I text back, my stomach sinking. Have I been so deceitful?

> *Well I think I would wanna know if that was the plan of the person I was starting to get to know, so at least I'd know early on where they're at in their life. 3rd date, 5th date, there's not that much of a real difference. I think it's important to mention.*

For our third date I took Orson to this charming French bistro near my house. There aren't any menus, and all the food is written on the giant chalkboard walls. We get seated at the bar, which we both like, and—bonus—one of the people in the kitchen is a queer who gives us the "family" treatment, sliding us some homemade crusty bread slathered with burrata and herbs. As I'm spiraling, we both nervously pick at our food, alternately gazing at each other and giggling. We talk about Ryan Gosling and how hot he is.

"I'm not, like, attracted to him, really," they explain. "But I would really like some of his sperm."

I choke on a Brussels sprout with browned butter and sage.

"I'm sorry!" Orson leans over, their face contorted with concern. "Was that TMI?"

I swallow my vegetable and drink some lemonade. "No, no!" I sputter. "Totally not! I love TMI!" This is it, this is it! I should tell them! *Speaking of Ryan Gosling's sperm, I'm going to try to get pregnant in a couple weeks!* But it seems like an awkward place to tell them, hemmed in by fellow diners, the generous queer fixing a cocktail in front of us. Maybe Orson would like a bit of privacy, to have their feelings? A moment to even figure out what their feelings are? A lot of masculine queer girl-boy people get really grossed out by sperm and penises and all that. I've known some who find the thought of their girl getting knocked up by some cis guy super threatening. Who knows what they'll say? Maybe I don't want to hear it here, at one of my favorite cozy bistros?

"Ryan Gosling's sperm," I cough out, "would be totally great sperm." And we're back to blushing and fidgeting and making each other laugh and falling into the vortex of *possibility and emotion* that are each other's eyes.

Back at my house, we're making out in my bed, and Orson is being a total champion about the fact that I am roommates with two feral cats found on the streets of Playa del Carmen even though they are allergic and forgot to take allergy medicine. In between the rolling around and the histamine sniffles is my building anxiety at everything I'm not saying. Finally, I can't take it anymore.

I blurt, "I'm going to try to get pregnant in a couple weeks!"

Orson does a double take, like in a movie. They shake their face quickly, snapping out of our dreamy make-out haze. Their eyes, which are like the New Order song that goes "Oh, you've got green eyes, oh, you've got blue eyes, oh, you've got grey eyes," get wide. I am distracted, totally swooning even as they are perhaps about to freak out.

"What? Are you serious?" they ask.

"Yeah." I start talking fast. "I mean, it's something I've been planning since the summer, and I just found a donor, and I'm forty, and if I don't right now, I might lose my chance, so I'm just going to do this, and I know this might be like really weird or freaky or fucked up to hear, and I'm sorry I didn't tell you earlier, but I just didn't know when to tell you."

"No, no." Orson slows me down. They're smiling. "No, that's . . ." They're choosing their words. "That's *awesome.*"

Awesome for you, I imagine their next words. *But I'm outta here! See ya!*

"I have some stuff in 'the vault,'" they tell me, sort of laughing. "My friend made me promise not to tell you right away, because she thought I'd scare you off, but . . . I really want to have a family. I really want kids. It's what I want more than anything."

"Are you *kidding me?*"

"No." They put their hands in front of them and get very serious. "I know this is your thing, I totally get that, and respect that, I'm just saying . . . I think kids are amazing. I'm really excited for you. Congratulations."

I put my hands on Orson, feeling around underneath their shirt for the circuitry board. They're an android, right? My friends, overcome with pity for my poor dating history, pitched in and had a *dream-date android* made for me. I am overcome with gratitude and love for my friends. They did such a great job! I don't even care Orson's an android! They're still one hundred percent more emotionally available than all my human dates!

But I find no circuitry panel, and when I bite their neck too hard, they say, "Ow!" I think they are real. But do they want to date a pregnant person? I'm going to start looking old really fast! I had been fortunate to pass for a thirty-something into year forty, but once that parasite starts sucking all the nutrients from my body, and once I start never sleeping again, I am going to look *old,* fast. I explain all this to Orson. "You'll keep dating me," I ask, "even if I'm pregnant and have really intense eye bags?"

Orson pauses. "Does this mean you want to keep dating *me?*"

"Yeah!" I practically scream. And we return to our make out.

6.

LOYAL AS A PIGEON

I have my first Insemination Plan laid out, and right away I see how my jet-setting lifestyle is going to make my complicated method of impregnation even more so. I've had standing plans to visit my good friend Gertrude out in Portland, and it so happens that the ovulation period I've been waiting for will happen while I'm there, six hundred miles away from Quentin.

But I've done my research. Under optimum conditions, sperm can live up to five days in a womb, with X chromosome sperm lasting the longest. Of course, a DIY home insemination isn't exactly optimum, but I arrange for Quentin to visit the night before I fly north, so he can provide me with some premium drag queen ejaculate. But, just in case it doesn't work, Gertrude arranges for a cis guy in her zine-making club to knock me up the old-fashioned way while I'm visiting. Old-fashioned—like, heterosexual sexual intercourse—*is* the optimum way to go, and I had made a pledge to myself that I wouldn't let any dating scenarios get in the way of my baby-making plans, so, even though I was probably falling in love with Orson, I was determined to get it on with this hopefully virile stranger while in Portland if all else failed.

Orson and I hadn't had *the talk* or anything—for all I knew, they were dating bunches of bitches who were trying to get pregnant! Even so, would they understand that this pending sexual activity was purely procreational? I kept the conversation about it brief, out of respect to the both of us. They seemed to get it. I felt relieved, but still worried: they were accepting of the situation, but would I be? I may not be strictly monogamy-minded, but I am as loyal as a pigeon and had bonded with Orson as my partner. When I stared deeply into their eyes, I would think, *I love you I love you I love you.* We were on the cusp of falling in love, when you already know you love the person but you just can't say it, because it's *crazy,* it's too *soon,* you'll *scare* them. So I didn't say anything, except telepathically.

THE NIGHT OF MY FIRST HOME INSEMINATION, I WAITED FOR RHONDA AND Quentin in my bathrobe with the blue and white stripes that looks like a beach lounger in Cannes. I felt romantic, dreamy, and excited. I'd picked a sprig of jasmine on my walk home and stuck it in a tiny glass bottle on my nightstand. I twisted the needle off an IV syringe I'd bought at Walgreens for fifty cents and set my oven to WARM and put a bowl in it. A bowl I once served candy and nuts in when I entertained. Did this mean I couldn't use it anymore, that it was forevermore the Sperm Bowl?

"I'm still going to use this bowl for snacks," I told Rhonda defiantly as we were obsessively scrutinizing Orson's Facebook page, waiting for Quentin. Rhonda agreed about the bowl. She had what she called an old-world approach to food and contamination. Like, she'd leave meat and dairy products out on the table forever and keep eating them. It didn't seem to hurt her, but Rhonda is an exceptionally hardy person.

Then, finally, there was Quentin! "Hiiiiii," he said, waving cutely. Quentin is *so adorable,* and since I'd last seen him, he'd grown a giant beard! It was chic and woodsy. Quentin has shiny, dirty-blond hair and big eyes and pouty lips and is just a looker. I felt myself developing an interesting crush on him. The crush a presently lezzed-out mother might get on her adorable fag sperm donor.

We discussed where Quentin should go to pleasure himself. It seemed the kitchen, at the other end of the house from my bedroom, would give him the most privacy. I escorted him into the small, brightly lit room. It had been a hectic day, and my sink was full of dishes. That was not very sexy. Two cat bowls sat on the floor, so I moved them into the other room, leaving a scatter of kibble on the linoleum. Mariah Carey was on my iTunes, and Orson's Facebook page was open on my computer.

"Um, do whatever you want," I said, and gestured. "You know, watch porn or whatever." I felt sort of bad presuming Quentin watched porn. There is something very wholesome about him— those big eyes, and how he works on political campaigns. I couldn't imagine him snorting a line or huffing a bottle of poppers backstage at the drag club. "I'm fine, I'm fine," Quentin kept saying, like he didn't want to put me out even though he was doing me the biggest favor ever.

Back in my bed, I positioned my hips on a stack of pillows. Like all lesbianish people, I had a giant unused box of latex gloves in my sex-toy box, just to show that I'd made the effort. I gave a couple to Rhonda, and we chitchatted until Quentin yelled, "Rhonda!" from the other room. In a panic, Rhonda leapt from the bed and slippery-slid out of my bedroom and into the kitchen. She returned holding the warm bowl nestled in a dish towel. "Okay, okay, okay, okay," she chanted. I held the bowl while she drew the sperm up into the syringe.

"Is it working?" I asked nervously.

"Yeah, yeah." She was focused on the bowl with that Scorpio-grade concentration. "I just want to get it all."

"Yeah, yeah, get it all!" I cheered.

Both of our hearts were pounding. I lay back and offered my bestie my vagina.

"Sorry," I said, apologizing for her having to see my genitalia like that.

"I don't want to hurt you," she said, carefully inserting the syringe.

"I'm fine!" I chirped. She pushed the plunger.

"We did it!" she cheered.

"Yay!" I hollered. There was sperm inside me, that's so weird! I swung my legs up in the air.

"The whole drive over I was like, 'I'm going to see Michelle's vagina, I'm going to see Michelle's vagina,' preparing myself," Rhonda said. "But then it wasn't really a big deal."

"Quentin, you can come in!" we yelled to Quentin. And thus began our ritual, to be repeated thrice monthly, as my ovulation is detected: Quentin in the kitchen, his call to Rhonda, Rhonda loading the syringe, me spreading my legs, insertion, insemination, letting Quentin know the coast is clear, and then a sweet and slightly awkward hang out, my friends standing around my bed while I lay there with my legs in the air. We giggled a lot, an ebb and flow of conversation that veered from normal, gossipy chitchat to suddenly reconnecting with the strange nature of our hangout and cheering on the drag queen sperm valiantly sashaying into my uterus.

We were together in a bright and special plot.

Eventually my team left, Rhonda home to bed and Quentin to the Occupy camp downtown. I pulled my gigantic Hitachi Magic Wand out from under my bed and gave myself an orgasm. It's supposed to help, I heard, though if a lady needed to have an orgasm in order to get pregnant, there would be no people. Right? Still, it's always nice to have an orgasm. I wrapped myself up in my robe and drifted to sleep smelling the jasmine on my nightstand. *If I get pregnant*, I thought, *I will press that jasmine and give it to my baby and we will always be able to smell a bit of the night they were conceived.*

A DAY LATER, IN PORTLAND, GERTRUDE WAS SCANDALIZED AND DELIGHTED THAT I'd have the sperm of two different men duking it out in my womb. "But how will you know who the father is?" she asked.

"We'll go on Maury Povich!" I imagined Quentin strutting on-stage in his drag persona, the crowd going bonkers. I had my practical, procreative rendezvous with Gertrude's friend, a long-haired zinester living in a punk-boy flophouse, Bikini Kill posters hanging askew on the wood-paneled walls of his bedroom. The next morning, a pee stick informed me that ovulation had ended, and I was relieved that a second round of sex with a strange zine man wouldn't be necessary, though he seemed like a very nice person. It's just too awkward to have utilitarian sex with a stranger, even for a higher purpose! I also felt unexpectedly connected to Quentin, invested in *him* being the donor, in having a little baby drag queen with a full beard and political convictions. It was so *Weetzie Bat!* And mostly I just didn't want to have sex with anyone but Orson. Before I left town, I told Orson, "I'm not dating anybody else. Just so you know." I needed them to understand that the scheduled fornication was *not* a date, and that there were no other dates. I wanted them to know everything. "Why would I date anybody else?" they said, and kissed me. The ease with which Orson just sailed us into a monogamous situation was unusual, and dazzling. So many queer people are drawn to explore more open situations; I myself am not immune to the lure of polyamory, something I've romanticized ever since I was a young person reading *The Diaries of Anaïs Nin*. But it felt so simple, so wholesome and cozy to take nonmonogamy—with all its instances of fording through jealousy and of epic processing sessions—off the table. It would be me, and Orson, and maybe, at some point, a baby, and really, what more did I possibly need?

7.

A BAD HOT DOG

Because it is the first time in my life that I might be pregnant, I begin to act as if I am. First step being cutting down my coffee consumption to one cup a day. This lasts for twenty-four hours, until I speak to my sister, who assures me I can continue to drink coffee until I get a pee stick positive for pregnancy. I can begin testing in about a week. There are all sorts of tests that promise early results, but I am determined not to be—in the words of the online Trying to Conceive (TTC) community—a *POAS maniac!* That would be a Pee-on-a-Stick maniac. The TTC community loves an acronym. My sister, who is, incidentally, trying to get pregnant with her second child, is definitely a POAS maniac. We call each other all day and compare our ovulation sticks. It's fun to be trying to get pregnant together! "We're like those teenagers in Massachusetts who made a pregnancy pact," she says.

A week or so after my Portland trip, my friend Sandwich comes to visit me from Eugene, Oregon. My plan is to convince her to move to San Francisco, but when I learn she is living in a Zen palace in the woods, with a hot tub and a redwood deck, *plus* having romantic intrigue with a straight girl who owns a horse, I give up. It is Sandwich, at my breakfast table eating yogurt, whom I announce my miscarriage to.

"Sandwich, I think I just miscarried," I tell her. She looks confused. "I just bled into the toilet, it was weird." Sandwich continues to look at me. Sandwich is a Libra, a gentle sort. Her style is neat and timeless, classy, but I think she is one of those reserved people who enjoy the antics of people who are more disgusting. I tell her about the reddish-orange splash of blood that fell into the bowl as I sat atop it. My period isn't due for nearly a week, but my period has become increasingly mysterious recently. Instead of coming on with terrible gusto, I spot for a couple days and then, nothing. Then—PERIOD! Wild, heavy, clotting, *Wombon* river rafting! I bleed through tampons, I ruin underwear! Then it's gone. All this willy-nilly bleeding has made it hard to know when to begin ovulation testing. And now this new blood. I do not know what to make of the little crimson splash.

I phone my sister, who knows everything about fertility, ovulation, pregnancy, and everything about my own personal pregnancy cycle, as she keeps better records than I do. Our mother has ceased to phone me for updates about my TTC goings-on and now calls my sister instead. I tell her about my bleeding.

"Well," she says, "it could be a lot of things. It could be implantation bleeding."

Implantation bleeding? What is *that?* Well, I find out, it is when your little fertilized egg finally reaches your womb, walks around a bit, rubs its finger along the countertop searching for dust, bounces a quarter off the bedsheets, decides the spot is up to par, and then hooks itself into your uterine wall with a teeny, tiny little barb that, despite its microscopicness, produces a bit of blood.

My sister has other fun information about bleeding while pregnant, such as the fact that some women bleed through their whole pregnancy and it's no big whoop. I am so happy I have not had a miscarriage, but decide to still work it with Sandwich and ask her to do everything for me because I am Implantation Bleeding, so I can't, you know, bring my breakfast dishes to the sink and whatnot. I also make her google "implantation bleeding" and read a result to me, even though it grosses her out a little. I disregard most of what it says, because actually it does *not* sound like I am implantation bleeding, but I want to be.

My sister phones me back. "I have to ask you a question," she says. "Don't think about it, just say yes or no, whatever pops into your mind first, okay?"

"Okay," I say.

"Are you pregnant?"

"Yes!" I squeak.

"I think you are, too," my sister says. "I could totally feel it when I got pregnant."

Okay, first of all, I have no idea if I am pregnant. None—nothing physical, nothing psychic, nada. I do not think I am like my sister; I do not believe I will just KNOW when I am pregnant. I think I am more like the women who have no idea they are pregnant and wind up giving birth in a Greyhound bus station bathroom, thinking they had only eaten a bad hot dog.

Still, I like that I *might* be pregnant, and I tell everyone, at an afternoon soul music dance party, "I might be pregnant! I might be pregnant! Isn't that wild?"

Orson arrives at the dance party, which is the whole point, to go soul dancing with Orson, and for Sandwich to meet Orson. "Not crazy" is Sandwich's immediate opinion of my newish paramour.

"I know!" I exclaim. "They're totally not crazy, right?"

"Yeah, they're normal," Sandwich confirms. I am overcome with joy. I finally am dating a normal person. That must mean that

I myself am almost normal. *And* I'm implantation bleeding. What a day!

Quentin arrives at the party, climbs onto a little pillar, and begins to go-go dance. "Look, look!" I grab Orson and Sandwich. "That's my sperm donor!" We coo over Quentin for bit, and Orson becomes obsessed with Quentin's adorable, punchy dance style. "He's got some moves!"

Orson has some moves, too. Orson looks like they just danced through a tear in the space-time continuum, like they started the evening dancing in a high school gymnasium somewhere in the Midwest, circa 1958, and wound up here, on the back patio of a dive bar, in a cluster of queers. It is our first time dancing together, and we both mention in a fake-casual way that we do *not* like to dance with other people. Like, we like to dance *around* other people, but we do our own thing. No touching. "No freaking," I say sternly. "I hate being freaked on the dance floor." Within a few songs we are all over each other.

It begins to rain, lightly at first but then hard, and no one stops dancing. I am splashing in a puddle, sure that my purse is lying in a pool of rainwater and spilled beer somewhere, but I do not care. Quentin has busted out a frilly pink umbrella and continues to go-go dance. Everyone is soaked, and the dance party takes on the energy of a wild celebration, like something remarkable has happened and we are here to mark the moment, rain be damned. I dance with my hands wrapped around my abdomen, like I'm dancing with my fertilized egg. I hope my dancing doesn't dislodge it! I try not to bounce too hard.

As it happens, I could have been slam dancing at the rainy dance party. My period showed me I was not pregnant, and my own investigation revealed that there hadn't even been a possibility of getting pregnant. Know why? I STOPPED inseminating when I got a positive-ovulation pee stick, but in fact that is when you are supposed to START inseminating! Now I learn that the ovulation tests look for the presence of ovulation-starting luteinizing hormone in your pee. When you get an LH surge, the egg is on its way! Time to get as much sperm up there as possible! That is not what I did. I instead called it all off, thinking my egg had plunked down in a nest of ejaculate and was hopefully being invaded. Duh! Doy! LaDoya Jackson!

I want to get knocked up while I am still forty years old. I just wasted a month, and now have only three or four months left. I buy another box of ovulation pee sticks and throw away that little sprig of jasmine, which my cats had stolen from the glass bottle beside my bed and were batting around the floor like a dead mouse.

I AM DUE TO VISIT MY SISTER IN LOS ANGELES THE NEXT MONTH DURING MY prime ovulation days. Like last time, I arrange for Quentin and Rhonda to visit the morning I fly to LAX, in the hope that if an egg tumbles out while I am visiting my sister, it will land in a cushy pile of sperm eager to make its acquaintance.

It is totally amazing to sit at my sister's kitchen table watching her intense fertility research skills in action. I am still wearing the winged menstrual pad I stuck onto my panties as I rushed out the door to catch my plane. There was no time for an orgasm after that morning's insemination, just some appreciative chitchat about Quentin's pink leggings ("I think they're Diane von Furstenberg"), a quick presentation of the new syringe (a squat, needleless syringe used to give babies oral medicine, given out for FREE at Walgreens!), the insemination itself, and then I was off to L.A., dribbling Quentin's precious, precious sperm into a pad the whole way.

"It takes sperm ten hours to reach the egg," my sister reads from her computer.

TEN HOURS. The more I learn about pregnancy, the more I marvel at how any of us are born at all. This should make me feel good about my odds, but I don't. It is easy for me to imagine that my body just won't *get* pregnant, though I try not to think of this because of everything we learned from *The Secret*.

My sister is ovulating this weekend, too. We go to Rite Aid together and pick up a couple packs of pee sticks, and the manager gawks at us while we use the self-checkout.

"Two friends getting pregnant," he observes.

"We're sisters," my sister corrects him.

"Well, I hope it works for you."

Last month, my sister went through seven pregnancy tests in three days. "If you ever want to buy stock, that's what you should buy stock in," she advises. "First Response. They're always going to do great."

My sister is insistent that I have an orgasm after each insemination. "'Orgasm helps the cervix dip into the vaginal pool and suck up sperm,'" she reads from a lesbian mom's post on the Berkeley Parents Network website. We both lose our minds a little over "vaginal pool." I imagine something like a Mexican cenote deep inside my body, with stalagmites and stalactites sparkling around my placid waters, sperm like those cave-dwelling blind fish darting through the blue. My sister is keeled over laughing. She's been very punchy for the past three years, raising a toddler, no sleep and lots of rhyming children's books and singsong. Sometimes something strikes her as hilarious, and she'll laugh until she's crying. It's great fun.

She then clicks over to a list of methods women once used to try to give themselves abortions: douching with a bottle of Coke, falling down a flight of stairs. None of them works. I take comfort in this. If these hardy little eggs can withstand getting fire-hosed by a carbonated beverage, maybe early life is not quite so fragile.

Truly, it's hard to know how to regard this endeavor. Pregnancy seems elusive, yet here we all are. About a quarter of all pregnancies end in miscarriage, and still, people keep getting born. My sister skims through various pregnancy sites, and I ask her to report on the font types and logos. "There are a lot of flowers," she confirms, pausing to scan a message board. "Oh, 'Cheeseburger Crotch,'" she reads, and collapses into hysterics again. "Do you know about Cheeseburger Crotch?" She wipes tears from her eyes.

My sister has a great monologue she occasionally launches into, called "They Don't Tell You." It's all the things no one tells you about pregnancy. Horrifying, grotesque things. She likes to share them, quickly following up each disgusting fact with, "But it's amaaaazing. Amazing." It's like a *Saturday Night Live* sketch about pregnancy. "Oh yeah, the stuff that comes out of your vagina, they don't tell you. It smells like DEATH, you have to wear a pad for a month, it just keeps coming and coming. But it's AMAZING. Amazing." Also, how you shit yourself and how they snip your taint. But it's amaaaazing. Pregnancy. Totally amazing.

"Michelle, your vag gets so big, it gets so gigantic, I guess if you were looking at it sideways, it'd look like a cheeseburger."

I just let that sit with me for a moment. This whole getting pregnant thing is a goodbye to vanity, I know. I can't get Botox while pregnant. I'll be left with "mummy tummy," abdominal muscles stretched thin enough to invite hernias. Fine. Now Cheeseburger Crotch. I accept this, and we move onto vulvar varicosities.

"Varicose veins in your pussy," my sister explains. We both explode into diabolical laughter. "And," she continues, "your nipples get really big and really dark and you look like the women in 1970s pregnancy and labor books."

My sister shuts her laptop, and I follow up on some text messages with Rhonda and Quentin, arranging for more insemination sessions upon my return. I decide it's time to invite Orson to the party. If I'm going to get serious about orgasms, I would appreciate their help.

8.

MISS SUPER EXTRA DELUXE PANDEMONIUM

When I come back from Los Angeles, Rhonda is waiting for me at the airport. We swing by Café Deeply Appreciative for a couple of fake mint chocolate chip milkshakes. Café Deeply Appreciative is a vegan raw food restaurant, so the chocolate chips are cacao nibs, which is like chewing on vaguely chocolatey splinters of wood. Rhonda is on a special diet of no gluten or cow dairy, so treats like these mean the world to her. Plus, she has not had an actual milkshake in many years and is happy with the facsimile. Afterward, we zoom to my house in her Honda Element, crammed with multiple skateboards, helmets, landscaping equipment, a stray branch or two, magazines, paper towels, sacks of gluten-free snacks, and the occasional bowl of oatmeal. It's insemination time!

This is a great insemination gathering because (a) it might get me pregnant! and (b) Orson is joining us for the first time. On the downside, I haven't gotten a positive pee stick for ovulation, and

I am concerned. But my sister said I had to do the insemination anyway, and so we all meet up at my apartment.

Quentin has a cold and is concerned about giving it to me via his sperm, but I never care about catching colds anyway. Orson, I learn, feels similarly—they just don't believe in catching colds. "I won't get it," they say dismissively when anyone is sick around them. They transfer this confidence to me. "You won't get sick," they say. "Neither of us will. We're too happy." I happen to super love magical thinking, so I decide that I'm too happy and in love with Orson to get a cold from Quentin's ejaculate.

While Quentin does his thing, Orson moves around my room, closing my blinds. This becomes their job at all inseminations hereafter. Orson is a Virgo and enjoys having a job. After Rhonda inseminates me, she leaves the room, and Orson turns the lights down and kisses me while I use my vibrator. I feel embarrassed in a way I don't normally feel when we have sex, like I have to make dumb jokes about the unwieldiness of the giant Hitachi or apologize for its deafening buzz. But Orson is a queer person and thus is not, you know, stunned by a Hitachi Magic Wand. It is very nice to have them there, as it is to have them anywhere, but especially at a moment so special. "Is this so awkward," I ask them, "that they're out there and everything?"

"No," they say. "I thought it would be, but it's fine."

It is interesting that everything the two of us think might be weird or awkward or gross winds up not actually being a big deal. Maybe it's because we're both children of chaotic families, skilled at integrating uncomfortable vibes. Maybe it's years and years of being queer: observing naked leather daddies at Pride; getting it on in gay bar bathrooms. Sexuality is less hidden, sometimes communal. Or maybe it's just the comfort we feel in each other's presence that puts everything else in the world on mute.

Soon we call Rhonda and Quentin back into the room, and I

lay alternately with my hips propped up on three pillows or doing a shoulder stand with my legs in the air.

"I got some on your floor," Quentin confesses, "but I wiped it up."

"Thank you," I say. Then: "Since entering my apartment, half of us have had orgasms." We laugh at this for a minute.

The next night, Quentin comes over wearing the most insane seasonal sweater I have ever seen. It is an autumn-themed seasonal sweater covered by a bunch of miniature autumn-themed seasonal sweaters. Quentin shared his concern that his sperm may not be up to par, due to tucking. Tucking, for the uninitiated, is what drag queens and assorted transgender ladies do to get their penis and balls out of the way. They tuck it all the way up between their legs and secure it there with, I'm not sure, bubble gum and twine, probably. Quentin worries that yanking and duct-taping his delicate sperm containers may have damaged his seed or reduced its potency. But Quentin is only twenty-whatever years old. I refuse to believe there is anything wrong with his sperm.

The next-next night Quentin arrives wearing a puffy vest and bearing donuts. We hang out on my bed with Rhonda and Orson, and it feels like a slumber party. We watch *Marcel the Shell with Shoes On* on Orson's iPhone. Then Rhonda and Orson start playing Words with Friends together on their phones. Rhonda plays the word *labia,* and I wonder if we should get started. I worry we are taking up Quentin's precious time—he's applying to graduate school in between drag shows and inseminations—but also, if we just get right to it, I worry he will feel used for his man-juice. It feels a little like managing a party, or an orgy—you want everyone to feel included and valued and have a good time.

After I'm inseminated and me and Orson have our moment, Rhonda and Quentin return to my room. Rhonda takes pictures of my feet in the air, because I am wearing black socks but my legs are naked, and this strikes everyone as comical. My insemination attire has remained my blue-striped robe, and Orson brings me a shabby chic blanket, which I wrap around myself like a diaper. Orson is very adorable, tucking the blanket all around so I don't accidentally moon Rhonda and Quentin. Orson is also very attentive to my temperature and never wants me to be cold. *What the fuck, Orson?* Are they trying to win a prize for being the nicest person in the whole world?

We try to figure out a good time to inseminate on Friday, a tough day for Quentin as he has a big Miss Super Extra Deluxe Pandemonium show that night. "Oh god!" I shriek. "Please, *please* come inseminate me as Pandemonium?" I beg. "Please!"

Quentin is not averse to absurdity—he is a drag queen, after all. I can tell he sort of likes the idea, but this time it's just not practical. "I could," he muses, "but I'm wearing a big light-up menorah. I don't think it would work." Quentin has a menorah costume that plugs into the wall, and each candle flame lights up individually, one at a time. Her head is the shamash, and she flicks her head so that it looks like the shamash is lighting all the others, per the tradition. Quentin is amazing. We decide that he can come over between his office's holiday party and his menorah drag prep, but he might be drunk. "That's great," I say. "A lot of people got conceived that way."

NOT THAT I EVER EVEN GOT A POSITIVE-OVULATION PEE STICK THIS MONTH. DID you know that some months you just don't ovulate? "If you're a girl, they don't tell you jack shit about your body," says my sister. I agree. I google early signs of pregnancy like mad, because things keep happening: I get a little nauseous in the back of a cab! Or, god, that body lotion smells disgusting—I must be pregnant! Nope, that body lotion just smells disgusting. Almond and ylang ylang? Bad call, Lush.

I fall into a fertility drug internet k-hole and decide to ask Sandwich to pick up a bottle of the oral fertility med Clomid while she's holidaying in Baja. God bless Mexico and its prescription-free pharmacies. Once, I came back from Mexico with a purseful of acyclovir, amoxicillin, Diflucon, and some amazing pink egg-shaped suppositories that cure bacterial vaginosis *and* yeast infections at the *same time* (what up, U.S.A., get competitive!). Also Viagra. The pharmacist totally judged me.

"Sandwich, will you get me Clomid in Mexico?" I figure she'll think I'm just joking, but Sandwich is so true blue, she totally hit the farmacia looking for fertility drugs. Sadly, she had gotten sick at the start of her vacation and passed out, into a metal gate, with her glasses on, so she had two big black eyes and was traveling with these bros who looked like frat dudes, and the pharmacists seemed to think she was a battered, kidnapped woman brought to Mexico to breed octuplets. "You want to *get* pregnant? Or you want to *not* get pregnant?" the pharmacist kept asking her, tenderly. "Maybe you want something for your eyes?"

Sandwich swung by San Francisco on her way back from Mexico, with no Clomid in tow, but with a super-tough-looking black eye. I guess sometimes it's fun to look self-destructive.

9.

FAIRLY FAMILIAR WITH MY VAGINA

Everyone is generously offering to amp up my fertility. A butch I've known for a while pledges to do a special Butch Fertility Dance in her home for me, some mystical moves that she swears have helped other women get pregnant. The Russian witch who cuts my hair in a salon that looks like an old-time forensics lab puts her hands on my belly and says something magical in her native tongue. Despite these efforts, I am not pregnant. My period comes, and now it's a tragic thing. When it arrives, people say "I'm sorry"—which on the one hand feels like a bit of justice, as if I've been waiting for SOMEONE to apologize for this monthly blood show ever since I got my very first menses at the tender age of twelve, in a fit of crying-hormones, while eating a box of Kraft Macaroni & Cheese. So, THANK YOU for the sympathy. But now, of course, my period signifies dashed hopes.

Presently, I'm annoyed and frustrated, haunted by the possibility that I might not even be fertile, despite the assurance of a fertility pee stick. I started out this whole process thinking: Win-win! If

I have a baby—win! What an adventure! If I can't have a baby—win! I go back to my totally amazing, routinely magical life, more magical now than ever before with the addition of Orson. But once you start doing something like this, it is hard to remain casual about it. It's hard not to get invested. And it's hard not to have feelings when your period comes.

The good thing about all this is that a few days into your period, it's time to get a new insemination plan together. I don't have time to shuffle about, sulking and eating hormonal bags of Jelly Bellys. I got work to do and a team at the ready.

My team, though, is heading south for the holidays. First, Rhonda will hop into a claptrap VW camper van with two skater bros (one, thank god, a Volkswagon van mechanic), one other lady, one twelve-year-old mini-skater, and one big dog. They plan to go to Baja, taking a scenic route that involves stops at crumbling, legendary punk houses with skate pools in the backyards and no toilet paper in the bathrooms. Soon after, Quentin will fly to Mexico City with a pack of gay boys. It seems that Quentin will be here for my fertile times, but Rhonda, carrier of the bowl, plunger of the spermy syringe, will be gone!

Before she leaves, Rhonda has a talk with me and Orson. It is very tender and thoughtful. She'd been thinking, now that Orson is in the picture, maybe I would want Orson to be the plunger of the spermy syringe. Of course, I had thought about Orson being the plunger of the spermy syringe. After all, they are my man, shouldn't they be knocking me up? But that's just not the way this has gone down, naturally, and though I don't know how much I care about natural *childbirth* (drugs and a C-section timed to give my child the optimal astrological chart seem like pretty cool options), I do like the way the Universe has arranged this sweet cluster of people to be here for me, and I want to keep them all! Everyone has their duties: Quentin barricades himself in the kitchen, a chair propped against the door to keep out the cats; I get Rhonda a pair of gloves while Orson closes the blinds; Rhonda grabs the bowl from Quentin; I hold it while she sucks the sperm into the syringe; she courageously faces down my vagina and then leaves me with Orson, who says hot, sweet things to me while I ride my vibrator. Everyone has a role.

Still, Rhonda will be on her skate trip soon, and Orson will need training. The plan shifts now to take full advantage of Quentin's generous spirit and get sperm up there every other day during my fertile period, bumping it up to every single day once I get a positive-ovulation pee stick.

Having learned much from all the romantic mishaps of my entire life, and having pledged to do things differently from here on out, I had made a pact with myself to *not* be the first person to say *I love you*. I am *always* that person, and have said it incorrectly on more than a few occasions, buoyed by intense brain chemicals, the kind that explode through your body during hot sex or, truly, even a particularly deep kiss. Having acknowledged the powerful feelings of love for Orson erupting in my body, I worked hard on keeping my mouth shut. Or, rather, keeping it open and full of Orson's mouth; it's hard to speak when you're all tangled up in a soul-kiss. Of course, I was telepathically expressing my devotion during those moments, in particular the seconds post-kiss when we stared intensely into each other's eyes. However, this could not go on forever. One of us would have to break, and truly, I have the astrological chart of a person prone to blurting *I love you*.

When I can no longer telepathically express my love, when I finally burst and say the words, they respond that they love me as well, and add the incredible flourish, "I'm going to buy you a house." This is absolutely the NICEST thing anyone has ever said to me, and the house that flashes in my mind is not a house at all but a château, a castle, so now I feel sort of like Cinderella, like I have to show that I am worthy of living in the castle. I can't FUCK IT UP by leaving spermy bowls around my bedroom. I resolve to be more tidy.

IT IS THE NIGHT OF ORSON'S IMPREGNATION TRAINING. AFTER QUENTIN HOLLERS, I hold the bowl and Rhonda demonstrates, pulling the plunger gently, sliding the nose of the syringe around the gloppy pool of semen. "I can smell it," Orson says, sounding surprised that semen has a smell, and that it's smellable. "Yeah, it has a smell," Rhonda agrees. I'm surprised, too; it's been a long, long time since I've been within smelling distance of sperm, and I've forgotten it has an odor. "What does it smell like?" I try to remember. I guess it carries a faint, earthy smell.

Orson is fairly familiar with my vagina, so that part is easy. Rhonda shows how to get the syringe in there and give the plunger a good smack. *"You want to shoot that stuff right up there!"* Even though it's all pretty simple, I can tell Orson is a little nervous. They're a perfectionist and want to do a really good job. They're so focused on their tutorial that they forget to close the blinds.

My team leaves for the night, and I am alone in my home, cats purring beside me on the bed. I discover that if I hang my head off the side of the bed I can really get my legs high in the air, to the point where I'm almost upside down! It seems like a really great way to get all the sperm running right into my cervix, until I lose my balance and flip backward off my bed—my nude vagina briefly in the air before my open blinds; a lamp, the empty sperm bowl, and a deck of tarot cards knocked off my nightstand—and land on my head on the floor.

MY WITCH, LULU TWILIGHT, SENDS ME A JAR OF HONEY, DECORATED WITH STAR anise and charmed with a fertility spell. Every modern woman should have a witch. It's a little like having a therapist, only there is less talking and crying on your end and more burning things and whispered incantations on their end. Lulu tells me to make a baby altar and talk to the Universe and ask them to send me a little person whom I can love forever.

Because I'm too busy to go to the witch store in the Mission, I grab my baby altar supplies at Walgreens and feel totally gross about it. Like—really? I'm making a magical baby altar to summon a special spirit into my body from the beyond, and I'm using a slightly glittered votive candle that smells like synthetic vanilla? I arrange my trashy Walgreens baby altar, placing a baby binky by the scented candle. My friend Daria had given me a stick of palo santo, and I burn that and scan my room for other items that could work on a baby altar, things that represent birth, fecundity, eggyness. A package of seeds from my friend who runs an urban farm? That's good. I sit before the altar and sip some Sleepytime mixed with the charmed honey, and ask the Universe to send me a person to love forever.

In the morning, I make a breakfast snack of an English muffin with peanut butter and charmed fertility honey. When I finish off the jar, I wash it out and place the scented candle in it. I rinse off the star anise that had been inside it and put that on my altar, too. A five-fingered star, like a tiny person's hand. The altar is totally coming together.

10.

SWIRLING ENERGY

Quentin shows up, and he's wearing the same striped wool cardigan that Orson has. My team inseminates in STYLE! I apologize to Quentin for the state of my house, like I usually do, and then I apologize for always apologizing for it. That must be annoying.

"I guess I'll just slip out the door afterward . . ." Quentin shrugs, this look on his face like he's choking on a giggle. It's a very mischievous look. Without Rhonda here, there is no one for him to hang out gossiping with while Orson and my vibrator and I have our ménage à trois. I feel sorry, or awkward, but Quentin assures me that he's into slipping out while Orson and I canoodle: "It makes me feel like your mother," he says, "which I like." Later, the door clicks closed behind Quentin.

Orson is sleepy; it's very late. They can't really sleep at my house ever, because the cats make their eyes swell and tear like they are watching the most tragic movie of all time, plus there is little actual sleeping at my house due to cats walking all over your head while you're trying to sleep, plus speed demons burning rubber under my bedroom window, drunkards hollering in the street, neighbors who perhaps cure their insomnia by playing video games, and the *plink plink plink* of leaky pipes inside my walls. Orson's apartment is so peaceful, set far back from the street, facing a garden with lemon trees and chickens. They kiss me goodbye and shuffle out of my house. I fall asleep feeling like a princess, hoping that deep inside my body a microscopic tadpole has busted into my cervix and is making the ten-hour swim to meet my egg.

THE PEE STICKS ARE MAKING ME CRAZY. WHEN I NOTICE THE LINE DARKEN EVEN a *little,* I get really excited and decide I'm ovulating, even though the instructions CLEARLY say that my pee line has to be *as dark or darker* than the control line. And it's not. It's just, like, a little darker, but I get all freaked out and amped like I'm ovulating, and start begging Quentin to come over every day, which he does, even though the holidays are now officially here and he is busier than ever. He arrives straight from a drag queen production of *The Golden Girls.* It appears that I will ovulate over the Christmas holiday, which is to be spent cooking food with Orson's friends and family and then watching all the *Twilight*s. Quentin comes over Christmas Eve morning, right *after* I burn a batch of Nestlé Toll House cookies and right *before* I shove a pear-cranberry crumble into the oven. Orson is already with their family, so I'm going to be inseminating myself. There is flour all over my kitchen, and greasy butter wrappers, and all I've eaten are some burnt chocolate chip cookies.

"How are you going to take your cobbler out," Quentin asks, "if you have your legs up for a half hour?"

Hmmmm. A valid question. I'll figure it out. "Why don't I put it in for you before I go?" Quentin offers. What a doll! *Oh hey, I'm Quentin, just stopping by to put a bun and a crumble in your metaphorical and actual ovens!* Amazing. (Later, he will confess to being stoned the night he came over from *The Golden Girls,* and the guilt prodded him to help out with the crumble.)

Quentin comes into my room and hands me the vintage cherry-red bowl of sperm. I suck the stuff up into the syringe, and it's sort of fun, like a game, a game of Get All the Sperm! I lie back and inseminate myself. I lie back for thirty minutes, kicking my legs up into a wonked shoulder stand, while the sugary smell of crumble seeps out of the kitchen and into my apartment. I love my team, but I have to admit that inseminating myself was pretty fun.

After the holiday, I get a special type of acupuncture that they give you when you hope you are ovulating. A row of needles across my belly. Needles in my feet, needles in my ears. I can feel a certain energy humming up inside me. It almost feels like being really turned on, but it's different than that. It's energy, swirling energy. "We're nourishing your uterus," the acupuncturist said, as she tapped the needles in. She'd also said, "I love making babies. The results are so visible." So many people seek acupuncture for subtle reasons, I imagine it's very satisfying to watch one of your clients come in with an ever-swelling belly. *I can't wait till I'm one of them,* I think to myself.

After one such session, back at Orson's, curled up on their couch watching *Once,* the energy in my lower abdomen is so electric, it's almost uncomfortable. I mean, it *is* uncomfortable, but it's exciting, too, because it means that acupuncture is real, it works, and this is the feeling of my uterus being nourished, this enduring, vibrating, almost ticklish sensitivity. It makes me wiggle on the couch, jostling Orson, who is sleeping because they tend to fall asleep when we watch a movie together.

"I Can Feel My Uterus," I whisper to them. *"It Feels Magical."* They open their eyes and kiss me.

11.

CATS LOVE IT
WHEN YOU'RE SICK

A few weeks later, Rhonda returns from her skate trip. We meet up at Café Deeply Appreciative to get bowls of tossed healthy things for dinner. The waitress brings us our bowls of kale and quinoa and seaweed with a smile and wipes her hand on her apron.

"Do you want to answer the question of the day?" she asks.

Sure, I say, with a twinge of resentment. It is ridiculous to feel resentment at Café Deeply Appreciative, because you know exactly what you are getting into when you go there.

"What are you creating?" the waitress asks us.

Rhonda and I look at each other. "A baby!" we burst in unison, and crack up.

My bowl comes with nori, which is good fertility food, and I get a drink called I Feel Better Now that has a shot of wheatgrass in it, which someone somewhere told me is good for fertility—I can't remember who, because every day someone gives me a new bit of information to toss onto my mental pile. I wash a mucus-thinning Mucinex down with my I Feel Better Now, to thin out any possible *hostile mucus* blocking the sperm from reaching the egg. No, Hostile Mucus is not the name of a queer, feminist band from the 1990s (though Ovarian Trolley is); it's a real term for a real phenomenon, when your cervical mucus gets so gelatinous, the sperm can't burrow through and instead expire from exhaustion. Tonight is the last insemination of the year. Each month my fertile period lasts six days, and by my calculation, this is my last fruitful day in December.

Earlier, on the phone, my sister praised me for doing such a good job "covering the spread," that nearly weeklong span of hopeful fecundity. "You really covered the spread," she says, and she continues to say this for the next week or so: "You did such a good job covering the spread." Earlier it was "You gotta cover the spread." Sometimes I think of my sister as a sports commentator on my conception efforts, up in her skybox, looking down, expert and opinionated. "Yes . . . there she goes . . . that's her fourth insemination on day fourteen of her cycle. I'd say she's doing a great job covering the spread. What do you say, Chuck?"

ON THE NIGHT OF THAT LAST INSEMINATION, I BUST OPEN A BOTTLE OF SPARK-kling cider and we all toast to the occasion. Quentin is leaving for his Mexico City adventure, and I am left with my body, which feels new to me now. Or, at least, I have never paid so much attention to it, focusing on every possible blip or wave of sensation. As someone who formerly claimed they were aware of having a body only while drunk or in the throes of sex, this fresh concentration is sort of fun. Is this what people mean when they say they're *grounded?* Look what an earth mama I'm becoming, and I'm almost certainly not even pregnant yet!

Or am I? I vow not to start with the pregnancy tests until the

DAY I am due for my period. I don't want to get on that obsessive train again. I just go about my life. One morning, I go out for breakfast with my friend Devin, who always says awesome, slightly non sequitur things. Like, "'Pump Up the Jam.' That was a groovy tune." Or, "When I think of women being witchy and reading tarot cards, I always think of that song 'Barracuda.'" On the way home, climbing the slight incline back to my apartment, I start to feel weird. Like I need to lie down right away. I say goodbye to Devin, heave myself up to my apartment, collapse on my bed, and call my sister. One of two things is wrong with me: I'm either pregnant, or I'm having Celexa withdrawal because too much sleeping at Orson's house has knocked me off my private bedtime ritual.

What *is* my private bedtime ritual? Pumice my feet and put on foot cream and socks. Read *Elle* magazine—oh, E. Jean! I love you!—maybe do some 12-step journaling if I'm "working a good program," and then I take Celexa, prenatal vitamins, DHEA, Coenzyme Q10, and a couple valerian. At Orson's, meanwhile, I don't even take off my makeup. Maybe I have forgotten to take my psych meds for, oh, like four days.

"Oh, sister, that's really not good!" my sister chides me.

"I know, sister," I agree. I can feel the dark storm clouds of free-floating doom and anxiety edging in on my wonderful life. I detail my symptoms. "Do you think I'm pregnant?"

"You could be," my sister muses. "But you could be coming off Celexa! Just spend the rest of the day in bed, can you do that?"

I spend the rest of the day in bed, reading *Elle* and text messaging, with cats on my lap. Cats love it when you're sick. By nighttime, I'm feeling normal again and go to Orson's house. I think it was just the Celexa, but now I really need to know, as does my sister, so I start with the pregnancy tests again.

When Orson gets up to walk their little dog, Rodney, a fluffy white thing with button eyes and a deranged personality, I slip into the bathroom and pee on a stick. I go back to bed. Later, when

Orson wakes me with coffee, I tell them I'm not pregnant. I tell them like it's this little detail, not a significant piece of information, an aside. Like, *Oh, Rodney left his dog toy in the bed. Oh, and by the way, I'm not pregnant.*

"Will you do your tests when I'm here?" Orson asks. "Will you let me know you're taking them, so I know right when it's happening?" I'm embarrassed at what a cowboy I am. It didn't even occur to me that Orson would want to BE THERE with me and SHARE THE EXPERIENCE with me, because they LOVE ME. I already know I have the tendency to take self-sufficiency to absurd, dysfunctional heights. It's nice to get called down from it.

The next morning, I tell Orson, "I'm going to pee on a stick." I pee on the stick and get a single, lonely line. "Not pregnant!" I yell from the toilet. I feel less vulnerable delivering the information thusly. I crawl back into bed, and we cuddle. In another day, I get my period. The intensity of the disappointment that floods my body is a shock. I had started this getting-pregnant project determined to graciously accept any inability to actually have a baby, but the feelings that accompany the surge of blood in my underwear are not so mild.

12.

THEY'RE A THEY

How, when I swore I would *not* resort to artificial baby-making procedures, did I come to be huddled in a doorway in the Marina, on the phone with a fertility clinic?

Okay, well, how I came to be in the Marina is fairly simple: I was at a 12-step meeting. You would think that a 12-step meeting in the Marina in San Francisco would be full of ladies with blowouts talking about how they bottomed out on white wine, and it is, but it's also a hotspot for individuals celebrating thirty days clean from crack cocaine and other folks fresh out of treatment programs. It's a real mix of people from divergent backgrounds, all cuddled together in a pale pink room, bonding over how we used to be THAT CLOSE to dying or going crazy and now we're all—comparatively—okay, and grateful. So, that's how I came to feel at home in this famously bourgeois neighborhood. But—talking to a fertility clinic? How did that happen?

A day earlier, I sat on my front stoop, on the phone with my sister, who was combing the internet for yet more information about these mysterious Intrauterine Inseminations. "You can do it," she kept saying. "From what I'm seeing, I think you can afford it." As a formerly poor person spawned from generations of broke people, I have a schizoid understanding of what I can or can't afford. I have savings, but aren't you supposed to save them? Isn't that why they're called "savings" and not "spendings"? As for my "spendings," why am I comfortable dropping a cash bomb on eye cream and anti-aging face wash at Sephora, but balk at spending money on, say, the dentist? Or a fertility clinic? If you don't crack into your savings for something as precious as a BABY, aren't you just hoarding money? Not that I'm against hoarding money—it sounds like something rich people do!

After months of investing in this pregnancy project, and with the additional motivation of having a family with Orson, I've become increasingly determined. I used to think fertility clinics were for desperate yuppies who needed to accept that they are barren women and move on with their lives, perhaps traveling the world and buying couture—something I always thought was a fine substitute for a baby. But that was before I was part of the TTC community. Once you set your mind on having a baby, an Alexander Wang bag is a cold consolation.

While browsing the designer clearance boutique around the corner from the 12-step hut, I suddenly "come to" before a rack of somewhat discounted Phillip Lim. My priorities are skewed! Or, at the very least, they are not helping me accomplish my Number One Goal, having a baby! I dash back out into the windy Marina, teetering on a pair of deeply discounted Mark & James platform pony pumps (see? See what I mean?) that I can't actually walk in—maybe because they were not made to be walked in but to be worn whilst reclining in a throne held aloft on the shoulders of some big, strong, shirtless men—where I huddle in a doorway and call the number for the fertility center. A lady answers the phone.

"Hi, I'm interested . . . in your services . . ?" Why do I feel like I'm calling a hooker? Because so many men ejaculate there?

"Okay, would you like to come in for an appointment, or would you like a phone consultation?"

"Um . . ."

"A visit is three hundred and seventy-five dollars but includes initial ultrasounds, and the amount gets deducted from your fees if you continue on with us. A half-hour phone consultation is free."

Three hundred and seventy-five dollars! That's half of a half-off Alexander Wang bag I could maybe find on sale somewhere! The obsessions of my former disinterested-in-motherhood self are hard to shake. "I'll take the phone consultation," I say, diving in.

"Okay . . . Can I have your name? . . . Okay, and your spouse's name?"

My *spouse?* Fairly presumptuous for a San Franciscan sperm bank! "Uh . . . Orson Kogan."

"Do you have insurance?"

"Nope."

"And your spouse, does he?"

"They're a they, Orson is a they," I say. "And we're not married," I add. Oh god, I hate this so much already.

"Okay, so you'll be requiring sperm as well."

"No, I have my own," I say.

"You . . . have sperm?"

"I have my own donor. I don't need additional sperm."

"Okay . . . I'm going to send you and Orson some online paperwork, and Dr. Evangelista will call you in two weeks at nine A.M. Please have the paperwork completed in advance of your consultation."

"Okay." I hang up and stand there teetering in my heels in the Marina, a great place to have an attack of low self-esteem, followed by an attack of fierce self-protective anger at being provoked into low self-esteem at the hands of a fertility clinic receptionist or, rather, the larger cultural/social/political systems we are all entrenched in all the time. It only takes a three-minute phone call outside my sweet queer bubble to come up against it. The feeling in my body is the same feeling I have felt, historically, while trying to get an apartment, a job, browsing at a high-end boutique, entering a fancy restaurant, meeting wealthy people whose money I want, meeting people's parents, when in close proximity to police officers, and so on. On most of these occasions I no longer get the creepy, dirty, impostorish, *I'm gonna get busted for something,* low-class blues. I now hang out at Barneys so much, certain sales people recognize me. Since getting sober, I am pretty much never breaking any sort of law, so add that to my white privilege and a nearby cop doesn't make me sweat. But I guess I can add fertility clinic to the list of experiences that make me feel shaky.

That night I learn, again, that I'm not pregnant. The main feeling I have at having to start scheduling another round of inseminations is dread. I continue to feel slightly bad about hitting up Quentin, like any minute he is going to rebel and take back his body. I fear that he is *so* over it but doesn't know how to get out of it. I don't like asking anyone for anything, and I'm not sure how I should check in with him about this. I don't know if he realized, when I asked him to be my donor, that this was something that could take years. I didn't. At what point do I throw in the towel and revert back to my other life plans—continue being a wild and eccentric, childless female, traveling and having affairs and splurging on avant-garde fashion? Those plans feel a lifetime away now. This whole process—taking a chance, finding myself bonded with Quentin, falling in love with Orson, and seeing that I didn't have to do it alone, I could have a partner, a family—it's changed me. Going back doesn't feel like an option anymore. My hope that Quentin won't mind sticking in for a few more rounds feels like a prayer in my heart as I fall asleep.

2012

THE IN/FERTILITY INDUSTRIAL COMPLEX; OR, INTIMIDATION

1.

SADSVILLE

Orson and I get along so well it might be a little bit disgusting. From the moment we first bonded about how shitty and mean our exes were over pie at a pie-centric restaurant on Church, it seemed like we regarded each other as discarded treasures, unjustly mistreated, unappreciated, our preciousness unseen. It would be our jobs to treat each other with love and dignity and fairness, partly because it's just how we rolled, but also to make up for the cruelty we'd each experienced. But I guess all couples have fights, even perfect couples like me and Orson.

THE SCENE: My bedroom. Orson is lying down, very tired from their day at the office. They also have PMS, but I don't know this!

THE TIME: 10:30 P.M. Rhonda and Quentin are both late for insemination, and texts keep rolling in warning that they'll be even later. This is stressful to Orson, who at the end of the hour-long Insemination Celebration will have to go home and walk Rodney before finally falling into bed.

THE FIGHT: Get ready to want to stab yourself in the cervix from boredom. Like all couples, we are about to fight about NOTH-ING. The outdoor soul party we love was throwing a legit *ball* at a campy ballroom by the sea in Santa Cruz, an hour or so away, and we, along with a gaggle of our friends, were going. I thought we'd drive out with their bestie, but Orson thought we were going with *my* bestie. My confusion confused and overwhelmed Orson! Their Virgo vigilance toward helpfulness, responsibility, and organiza-tion struggled beneath an oppressive cape of exhaustion and PMS! Orson, whose speaking tones are always laden with butterflies and honey and kittens in baskets, SNAPS AT ME!

As I pet them gently, cooing, "Don't worry, I'll sort it out," Orson stops my hand and says, "Don't do that, it's condescending."

I actually think they're joking, like how they sometimes turn to me sternly in a public place and say, "Do I know you? Why are you following me?" They will also sometimes just run away from me in the street for no apparent reason. I love these jokes! So, upon my bed, I freeze and say, "Huh, whaaaa?" with a crooked smile on my face.

"I don't like that," Orson snaps again. "It feels condescending."

Butterflies fall from the sky. Hives of honey dry up as bees die. Kittens tumble from their baskets.

"I'm sorry," I think I say. "I didn't mean to be condescend-ing." I flop down on top of them like I've been shot, burying my head in my pillow so they don't see that I've immediately begun to bawl, because inside I am about five years old and burst into tears whenever anyone speaks to me harshly. I lie there until my doorbell rings. Thankfully, now that I'm on meds, I can actually *stop* cry-ing once I start, unlike the unmedicated years when I would just have to lock myself in the bathroom for about four hours until the sobbing subsided, and then need to smoke a pack of cigarettes to maintain my fragile equilibrium.

By the time Quentin and Rhonda walk into my apartment, I'm

composed, though my face looks red and puffy, like I just woke up. I stretch and yawn and make a performance of how I'd fallen asleep. Nothing feels worse than covering up a fight with a lie, but I'm still shaky and I don't want to deal with it. I want to get inseminated and get my friends out of my house so I can burst into tears again.

After Rhonda shoots me up, Orson and I lie side by side in my bed. We just lie there, not talking. We're in a fight! What will happen? How does Orson deal with fights? How do I?

Traditionally, I've had two conflict responses in my relationships. The first: respond in kind. I get all high and mighty, like, I Will NOT Be Spoken to Like That! Alternately, I burst into my aforementioned sobs and am a martyr about it. But I don't want to do either with Orson; that's not our energy.

After lying there for a moment, I call for Rhonda and Quentin, who bound in excitedly. Rhonda pushes Quentin to share with us the story of his first childhood talent show, when he Rollerbladed to Cyndi Lauper's "Time After Time" in a pair of leopard-print capri-length tearaways. This lifts my spirits for a moment, but then they leave and it is back to Sadsville.

"Do you want to talk?" Orson asks, and I start crying again. I've been in relationships where I was spoken to in crummy tones like that all the time, and it was awful. I think part of me is afraid that I've crossed some sort of threshold with Orson—like maybe my novelty has worn off and now I'm just someone annoying to snap at for the rest of our lives together.

"Do you still like me?" I ask pathetically.

They drape themselves over me in a full-body hug. "Like you? I want to marry you!"

Well, this sure makes me feel better immediately! Though I am sure I will obsess about this statement for the foreseeable future, I promise myself I'll never, ever mention it. It's not a proposal. It's a sweet, honest, and desperate blurt from Orson, who is now also crying!

"I never want to make you cry!" they say, tears streaming from their eyes.

"I never want to be condescending or hurt your feelings!" I cry back. We kiss our teary faces. Orson brings me a pint of Three Twins Mint Confetti ice cream from my freezer, so I don't get up and disturb the sperm. They kiss me good night and leave for home, sending me love texts along the way. I eat the rest of my feelings and fall asleep under a pile of cats.

The next morning is my phone consultation with the fertility clinic. I wait and wait for a call from Dr. Evangelista, and after fifteen minutes I call the clinic myself.

"Oh, your appointment has been canceled," the receptionist tells me.

"What?" I ask. "But why?"

"You never filled out the information on our web page," the woman tells me. "I left you three messages about it." She sounds annoyed, and I feel a surge of defensiveness. But the reality is, I don't answer my stupid phone. My voice mail is very neglected.

"Your website wouldn't let me move forward," I protested. "I couldn't get to the intake!" I realize, as I begin to cry, that I'm still feeling fragile from the night before. Emotions! I make another appointment with Dr. Evangelista and hang up. I also pee on a lot of pee sticks, because I just can't tell if my pee line is as dark as the control. I take a picture of the latest pee stick and text it out to my team. *AM I OVULATING YET OR WHAT?* I ask. The consensus is no, but that's not going to stop us from inseminating, because we are going to COVER THE SPREAD!

2.

HOW MUCH DOES
THIS SHIT COST?

My sister visits me from Los Angeles, accompanied by the tiny fetus growing in her belly. Madeline is pregnant!

When she first found out she was preggers, Madeline was afraid the news would make me sad or upset. But I am only excited for my sister, the source of all fertility information, tracker of my period. It seems only right that she would get pregnant sooner, as she is the master. And now I get to have another niece/nephew person!

"Are you sure you are okay?" I am sure! If anything, it is proof that it happens—people get pregnant! I am a person, therefore I may get pregnant, too!

Before my sister leaves town, she confers with me about Orson.

"Orson is *amazing*," Madeline says, her voice full of wonder. "Do you know what they did at pancakes, when you went to the bathroom?"

Apparently, Orson leaned across the table and said, "I really like your sister," in this earnest, sincere way.

"It was so . . . old-fashioned!" Madeline exclaims, delighted. "No one has ever done anything like that before!" She is nodding in approval. "This is the one."

I get a luteinizing hormone surge on Monday, meaning I could ovulate at any minute. Monday is also the day of our reservations at the motherfucking French Laundry, for Bernadine's birthday. We've had these reservations for months, because it takes months to get them. Which is handy, because then you have time to save up/come around to accepting that you are about to spend THREE HUNDRED DOLLARS on dinner. Our reservations are early, and the drive north is long, so Quentin graciously comes over on his lunch hour to knock me up. I pull my satin and leather dress above my hips, and Orson inseminates me. I have my tights and booties waiting right beside me so I can just fly out of bed and downstairs to the rental car.

How was French Laundry, you may want to know. In my opinion, the lobster was tough and not the butter-dunked delight I expect from a lobster, and the deconstructed Caesar salad clever but the chicken kind of gross. It is a heady, giddy experience to do something so luxurious that it feels transgressive. I can say that I ate at the French Laundry. Hey—I ate at the French Laundry! There's something I'll never do again, despite Bernadine's blissful calculations that if you never ate out anyplace else, and cooked inexpensive meals at home 364 days a year, you could actually dine at the French Laundry seasonally.

I am happy I did something so decadent before I have a baby and can never again spend money on anything that does not support the higher cause of my child's eternal happiness and success, I think to myself. That shining plate of puffy, cheesy gougères now takes its place in my memories, aside a pair of Rag & Bones jeans I will never again be able to fit into, nor justify replacing, once I am a mom.

Speaking of the spending habits of the upper class, it's time for my telephone intake with fertility specialist Dr. Evangelista. I wonder if she questions my commitment, as I selected the free phone consultation over the *put your money where your mouth is* three-hundred-dollar live consultation—*with complimentary ultrasound!* I'm just kidding about that. Nothing in this situation is complimentary. (Incidentally, the French Laundry does give you "complimentary" donut holes to dunk in an espresso cup full of semifreddo, *and* cellophane-wrapped packages of their famous shortbread, *and* a souvenir printout of your menu, so you leave feeling like you got a bunch of stuff for free, but you really, really did not.)

"Before we begin, are there any questions I can answer for you?"

Of course, there is really only one question: How much does this shit cost?

"An IUI cycle with Clomid will go between eight hundred to one thousand dollars; a cycle with human chorionic hormone is between twenty-five hundred and thirty-five hundred. Plus another fifteen hundred dollars in both instances, for donor screening."

My body fills so completely and instantaneously with dread, I'm a dread balloon. If it was a one-time thing, this expense, I'd do it. But IUIs often don't take the first time, and after making an eight-hundred-dollar commitment to go that route, what are you going to do when it doesn't work? You'll feel like you really wasted your money if you give up, even if, like me, you have but a 5 percent chance of getting knocked up.

I won't understand until later, when I talk to Madeline, that that 5 percent improves the more chances I take. As a forty-year-old, I don't have a static 5 percent chance; after four months, I've got a 20 percent chance, almost as good as a drunk twenty-something who forgot to make her hookup wear a condom. But I don't realize this until later, so my dread now morphs into a stunned numbness.

Just as my odds aren't static, neither is that $1,500 donor screening charge. If we run out of his sperm reserves, each additional deposit costs another $1,500.

It would be nice—really nice—if fertility clinics had customer-appreciation cards. Like, get nine IUIs and your tenth one is free? Two-for-one donor screenings? I ask Dr. Evangelista how much the odds increase by utilizing these procedures.

"At your age," the doctor summarizes, "you're at a critical point. The difference even between forty and forty-one is significant."

"Okay," I say.

"Any more questions?"

"I'm just going to, um, think things over," I lie. There is nothing to think over. I am not going to this, or possibly any, fertility clinic. I'd be better off taking my savings to Vegas and sprinkling the money over roulette tables.

"Okay, well, best of luck to you." *You're going to need it,* I imagine Dr. Evangelista cackling as she hurls her phone into the cradle. *Another impoverished, baby-mad hag gets her comeuppance!*

3.

LIFE'S BIGGEST ADVENTURE

So I'm really sad after talking to Dr. Evangelista. I liked knowing there were some options if home insemination gets too frustrating, but now those options don't really feel like options. But maybe I just need to let the price sink in for a while. Sometimes you just have to warm up to what something costs. When I first found out how much a KitchenAid mixer costs, I was angry at the world about it. I really wanted one of those colorful, shining appliances sitting on my countertop, but they're like two hundred and fifty dollars. Two hundred and fifty dollars! It was a wonder that anyone had one at all! After the shock wore off and I had come to accept that two hundred and fifty dollars is what a KitchenAid mixer goes for, I found one on sale at a kitchen outlet for one hundred and seventy-five dollars. Now, a one-hundred-and-seventy-five-dollar mixer is not cheap, but compared to two hundred and fifty dollars, it was a bargain, so I jumped on it, and even got an additional 10 percent off for buying the floor model. I doubt I am going to stumble across a fertility outlet shop, but there is still a lesson here. Sometimes a price that at first feels upsettingly expensive turns into just what something costs. It becomes normal. And then you're a little closer to having it.

My sister tells me about a test she needs to have to check on the genetic health of her own gestating fetus. Her doctor insisted that she double-, then triple-check that her insurance covered it, because if she paid for it up front it was five hundred dollars, but they bill insurance companies three thousand dollars. If her insurance company balked, she'd be stuck with that astronomical bill. "Why?" Madeline demanded—not of her doctor, but of me. "This is why health care and health insurance in this country is so fucked. Why are there two different prices?"

Madeline asks me if my conversation with Dr. Evangelista made me sad, and I tell her it did, pushing myself to be honest and vulnerable, even though I am most comfortable in my It's Cool, I'm Indomitable and Optimistic and Nothing Gets Me Down persona. It's so *vulnerable* to feel vulnerable.

"I'm sorry," my sister says, her voice laden with empathy. I had told myself that it would *not* be a tragedy if I couldn't get pregnant, but everyone being all tender and bummed on my behalf is getting in the way of that carefree attitude.

"There's always adoption if this doesn't work out," I tell her. And if I go that route, I get to bump my coffee intake *back up* to my preferred three to five cups per day. It doesn't sound so bad, really. But the urge to actually be pregnant, to feel a baby growing inside me, watch my body morph and shift, the urge to *breastfeed*—these are all real urges. I know I would be psyched to raise an adopted baby, but I'm not ready to let go of the dream of pregnancy.

THE MORNING AFTER THAT MONTH'S FINAL INSEMINATION, I WAKE UP AND USE the bathroom. When I wipe myself, the toilet paper slides over my parts like greased lightning. Cervical mucus! Great, shining gobs of it! I get on the horn to Quentin and ask if he can actually come over *again,* and then I make an appointment for acupuncture. On my way, I stop at the health food co-op and buy a big bottle of this German blood tonic one of the acupuncturists recommended visits ago. I hadn't gotten it—what was I waiting for? Why was I doing all this if I wasn't going to follow through on their advice? There it is on the shelf, gold-capped, the label decorated with berries, the glass of the bottle dark enough to obscure the disturbingly gory hue of the liquid. It's made from carrots and a shit ton of vegetables, but the iron tang of it is so meaty, I have to hold my nose when I take a shot of it three times a day.

At acupuncture, I can feel my heart chakra open up as I lie back in the recliner. A spinning throb in my solar plexus. I am full of love! Ready to give it and ready to get it. I try to talk to the baby-spirit in my head but get distracted thinking about other things and then worry that this means I don't want the baby enough and so it won't come down. I'm already a bad mother, and the Universe is going to punish me for it by not letting me become a mother at all! I know that if babies avoid being born to spaced-out women, there would be *far* fewer humans on the planet, but that doesn't stop me from feeling superstitious. This whole process is so far beyond my control, it's easy to obsess over the tiny places where I think I might have influence, even a mystical one.

Quentin asks if he can bring over the friend he's picking up at the airport. A stranger at the Insemination Celebration? Why not!

Quentin shows up with his old college friend Morgan. I can't tell if Morgan goes by *he* or *she,* so I avoid pronouns and instead just talk about how awkward it is that we're meeting for the first time under these circumstances. I learn that Morgan is also planning on using Quentin's sperm for a future baby. "Oh my god!" I gasp. "Our kids will be half siblings!" How wild! Morgan is drinking a beverage from a mason jar like someone who just hopped a train from Portland. I learn about how Morgan thought Quentin was *straight* when they first met at Brown, which is truly mind-blowing. Morgan and I chat while Quentin does his duty in the kitchen, and then I kick them both out of my room and do my own duty, and then I call them back into my bedroom and we end up in a passionate conversation about what is and what is *not* Italian ice or, what we called it where I'm from, *slush*.

Slush is my most favorite treat, and I am very opinionated about it. Slush is not a Slush Puppie—a Slush Puppie is a grossly sugared liquid beverage with a bunch of ice sloshing around in it. Also, shaved ice is not a slush—shaved ice is a bunch of snow with sugar syrup poured onto it, melting half the snow in the process. The little cups of Italian ice you find prepackaged in some stores, the kind you scrape with a wooden spoon, those are cute, and I enjoy them, but they are not slush. I don't know how slush is made, but it gets scooped from a bucket like ice cream does: a dense cup of tightly packed snow that tastes like lemon or raspberry or watermelon. In Boston, they sell it in convenience stores or out of carts on the Boston Common; in New York, most pizza places have it. In the entire state of California, there is only one place to get this, my favorite treat—a shop on Melrose in Los Angeles, operated by folks from Philadelphia. There are some fancy restaurants in San Francisco that sell granita, the high-brow Italian version of slush, but it just isn't the same.

Morgan wants some restaurant recommendations, and I tell them to go to Acquerello if they want to spend bank, not to miss Mission Chinese Food or brunch at Mission Beach café, and, yes, I think buying a rotisserie chicken at Zuni and having it for lunch all week is an excellent idea. "I am not backing down this year," Morgan says cryptically. "This is the year to go all the way." Right on, man! Before they leave, I make a plan for Morgan to take my cats once I'm knocked up. If all goes well for both of us, we will someday be family.

LATER THAT WEEK I MEET UP WITH MY OLDER WRITER FRIEND CANDICE, THE ONE who told me to get the FSH test back at the start of this wonky journey. We convene at the fake French café near my house. Candice's butch girlfriend had their baby for them about eighteen years ago, and he's now this tall, adorable boy with a head full of wild, golden curls, attending some cool college, and he's *gay!* Another older lez I know tells me her son is gay, too. I'm sure gays who are trying hard to make everyone think they are totally normal and just like straight people won't like this claim, but I bet that gay people are more likely to have gay kids. Maybe in part because of some neat queer gene, but also because *I* think a lot more people would be a *lot* more gay if they knew it was an option. Being raised in a home where it's super awesome and no big whoop to be gay probably makes more people feel relaxed about their gayer impulses. Just a theory! What do I know? I've heard that Randall Terry, the creep who started Operation Rescue, was raised by lesbians, so I could be horribly wrong.

Candice has the *best* stories about her girlfriend, Jessie, having their baby. How Jessie rode a motorcycle till she was seven months pregnant ("Eight months," Jessie proudly corrects me when I run into her at a poetry reading). How the influx of hormones a pregnant woman is bombarded with includes testosterone, and so Jessie got super buff. How she wore her leather motorcycle jacket open over her giant preggers belly.

Candice thinks it is so cool that I'm trying to get knocked up. "Having a baby puts you in life's biggest adventure," she says, and I believe her. I am all about adventure! I like her attitude. "Your values change," she says, "but they change slowly." Like how it took Candice and Jessie a moment to realize a crystal meth enthusiast was not an appropriate babysitter. Or how they surprised themselves by *insisting* their son go to college.

I can't foresee how my values will change once there is a baby in the picture, but I think I'm down with it, whatever it looks like. It's ridiculous to expect that such a life-changing experience *won't* change you. When I first got sober, I thought my life would stay totally the same, I'd just take the booze out of it. This is one of the sillier thoughts I've had. My life changed *entirely,* and when I stopped resisting it, I realized that the changes were one hundred percent for the better. So I let it change, and I changed, too. Nine years later, everything is way cooler than I could have imagined back when I was desperately trying to keep hanging out with drug-addled people in the boozy environments I was terrified to let go of. I like who I am without booze and dive bars, and I'll probably like who I am with a baby and all the unknown mommy concerns that come with it.

A week or so later, on the toilet at my gym, I am greeted by a splotch of blood in my underwear. Goddammit. I begin texting my sister from the bowl. *What color blood is it?* she asks, ever-hopeful for the elusive implantation bleeding. We go back and forth about the exact shade and hue of the stuff in my underwear, trying to Sherlock if it's my period or something better, but I know in my gut it's my period. I send a text to Orson, who is home sick with a cold (see? Happy people *do* get sick), and they text back that they wish they were snuggling me.

On the bowl, inspecting the crotch of my drawers, the desire to take the matter of my fertility into my own hands intensifies. I'm sick of these periods! I need to get me some Clomid. As a former drug addict, I refuse to believe I can't score whatever chemicals I want. I shoot a text to my friend Dirk, a rent boy who orders bulk Viagra on the internet. *What dosage?* he asks. *How many? Um . . .* I text back. *Not sure how many, but the highest dosage!* Right? I want this shit to work! *I'll send you an email in five minutes,* Dirk texts.

I arrive home to multiple emails from Dirk, messages that come from an unfamiliar email, clearly his hooker account. I email with him while texting with my sister, who is simultaneously on About.com researching Clomid.

If you say that your order never came they'll send you another package, so you get two batches for the price of one, Dirk, an expert scammer, advises. *It doesn't always work, tho.*

But how much Clomid do I even need? According to the texts coming in from Madeline, I take five per cycle. This website sells them in bundles of thirty, so I'm already set for six months with a single purchase. I can't imagine I'd need more than that. If these shady drugs don't hook me up with a belly full of triplets or at least a good set of conjoined twins within six months, I think it's time to move on to the harder stuff.

This website offers free Viagra with a purchase of fertility meds. I text this amazing bonus to my sister. I wonder if I'll give it to Quentin or save it for myself? Viagra works for girls, too! My sister sends me a text insisting that I should only get the 50 milligram Clomid, not the 100 milligram. *God, I'm such a drug addict,* I text her. The kind of drug addict I am is: if a little is good, a lot is better. I change my dosage on the website and the price drops by ten dollars. A thrill shoots through me. *It's cheaper,* I text my sister. This cracks her up, so I start texting her phonetically in the accent of our homeland, the North Shore of Boston. *Wicked pissah! It's a sawbuck cheapah!*

A text from my sister flashes on my phone. *How is this even possible? That you can just order drugs over the internet?*

I have no idea, I text back. *All I know is you can, and it's coming from India.*

Madeline texts me everything I need to know: I take the Clomid on the fifth day of my period, and I take it for five days only, at the same time of the day. Side effects include nausea, mood swings, hot flashes; if I get blurry vision, I should call a doctor. I enter all my information into this shady website; later, I will wonder if this is how some miscreants tried to charge $5,000 worth of computer equipment and gaming time on my card. Five thousand dollars! That's like four Clomid IUIs!

Days after finding blood spots in my underwear at the gym, my period has not really come on. It's just—spot, spot, spot. *Maybe it's not your period,* my sister nudges hopefully. *Take another test!* I find myself in the odd situation of beginning my morning with two different pee sticks: one to track my ovulation, just in case this *is* the fifth day of my period, and then a pregnancy test, in case it's not. Both of my tests come out negative. My underwear keeps getting soiled with bits of drippy, brownish blood, and I can feel the unspoken hope of everyone around me.

One night Orson returns from walking Rodney with a perfect, dead hummingbird cupped in their hand. It's amazing to see a still hummingbird. Its feathers are sleek and iridescent. There isn't a mark on it, as if its wild little hummingbird heart stopped beating and it just fell from the sky. Orson buries it while I shower and try not to narcissistically make the tender hummingbird's death into some sort of omen for my condition. Hummingbirds are one of my familiars. I feel certain I'm not pregnant. Soon the blood dripping from my body surges, confirming this.

My friend Dirk, the Viagra-popping rent boy, lets me, Bernadine, and Tali use his vacation cabin in the woods for a work retreat. In addition to being a rent boy, Dirk is also a witch, and he tells me one of the rooms in the cabin is dense with fertility magic. A close friend of his has been trying to get pregnant in it, and so he had been casting the room with vibrations and energy, making it the perfect place for me to stay. The room does feel great, but Dirk's whole cabin does, because he and his boyfriend, Coyote, are such lovely, spell-casting fairy faggots. At night I sleep among African fertility goddess figurines. In the morning I get another "?" ovulation stick, plus a text from my sister that she is having a boy. I know gender isn't real, but it's still exciting!

Back in San Francisco, Orson and I head toward the witch store in the Mission to buy a DivaCup, which I had read on a message board could help with the insemination process. I didn't expect it to be so *big*. It also comes with a branded lapel pin, which kills me. First, *diva* is right up there with *rock star* under phrases I wish to never hear again. I mostly find it hilarious that the makers of a cup meant to CONTAIN MENSTRUAL BLOOD think that their customers would want to advertise their choice of menstrual blood containment with a bit of jewelry. I'm all for killing the stigma of menstruation—in the nineties I ran a grotesque little personal experiment that involved my simply not wearing ANYTHING when I got my period and bleeding all over the place to make people DEAL with the fact that WOMEN MENSTRUATE! That was during one of the more extreme peaks (valleys?) of my Lesbian Feminist Nervous Breakdown. So I'm down to dismantle patriarchal period shame; I just don't know that a lapel pin that says DIVA is the way to do it.

The sales witch shows me that there are two different sizes, one for women who are over thirty or have had kids, and one for younger women or women who haven't.

"I'm not really using it for my period," I tell her. "I'm using it to help me get pregnant."

"Oh . . ." She looks at me with confusion. "You put it up there after you have sex?"

"Yeah," I said. To say anything else would force me to face my annoyance that this woman, working in an infamous lesbionic witchery shop in a pretty gay neighborhood (a) isn't up to date on the methods women (lesbians) may use to get themselves pregnant, (b) presumes her customers are straight, and (c) thinks Orson, standing handsomely beside me, is either a man or a straight girl or perhaps my younger brother. It's too much to grapple with. At the last second, I freak and decide against this message-board plan. Wearing a DivaCup filled with sperm feels too ludicrous, even for me.

Instead of buying the DivaCup, I buy a copy of Janet Spiller's *New Moon Astrology*, so I can get consistent with my new moon-wishing rituals. Soon it will be my birthday, and Orson and I will be going up to Northern California, to stay in the rustic Hotel Arcata. The Arcata has claw-foot bathtubs, and I want to get a fun bubble bath. We come across one of my favorite bath treats, a Love Spell Fizzy Melt by Apothekerri.

"Well, you're warned," I tease Orson, waving the love spell bath thingy at them. "If you get in the tub with this, you might fall in love with me."

To my confusion, Orson does not make a joke in return. They look . . . sheepish!

"What?" I ask them. "Why are you turning all red like that?"

"Well . . . I just . . . maybe, when we were first dating, I put a love spell on you?"

"WHAT?" I am utterly shocked. Orson is a very open-minded and openhearted person, but they also tend more toward the logical and rational than the witchy and woo. I am utterly dazzled, dazzled and charmed.

"Remember I went on that ghost tour with work, around Halloween?"

"Yes," I say.

"Well, at the end they passed around this, like, voodoo doll, and everyone made a wish on it, and I wished that you would fall in love with me."

"You did!" I remember where we were with each other around Halloween, how I was falling in love with them. Though there were things about us that didn't sync up, I felt doggedly driven to move toward them. Was it an enchantment all along?

"Babe, I'm sorry!" Orson looks seriously pained. "I don't want to put a spell on you!"

It's true that you shouldn't cast love spells, because they tamper with another's free will, though this is a rather new philosophy.

The history of magic in all its many traditions offers up many love spells. You just have to be prepared for the consequences, which in Orson's case means I'll be hanging around for the rest of their life.

"You're so powerful!" I exclaim. "I had no idea you were such a wizard! Or a druid! A Manwitch!" Maybe I should be disturbed that I've been spellbound, that this love I feel for Orson is possibly the result of occult tampering with my free will, but really I'm just giddy that when they were prompted to make a wish, I was what they wished for.

4.

ABOVE AVERAGE IN EVERY WAY

Jesus Christ, there are babies EVERYWHERE. And they are out with their dads. Cute, scruffy Mission dudes with babies slung all over them like messenger bags. The Mission is New Dad Central, and Orson and I look at them with a mixture of longing and inspiration.

"I can't wait for those weekends when you get to sleep in and I take the baby out for a walk," says Orson, already practiced at early-morning walks with Rodney. I could imagine this: getting to lie in bed in our home's sweet stillness, Orson out with the baby, both of them bursting back in a clamor, raising me from the bed. I just have to get pregnant and make it happen.

On the night of the next insemination, Orson can't be there. I'm busy, too, having been asked to speak at an artists' colony on the occasion of their thirtieth birthday. The colony is over in Marin, and, me being driver's license–less, they are sending a car for me! My younger self is in disbelief. I plan for Quentin and Rhonda to come over with just enough time to let me lie there with the sperm in me before running down to my ride. But the car service rings me twenty minutes into my insemination; they're right downstairs. "Uh, I'm going to need ten more minutes," I tell the driver, looking up at my legs, posed in midair. I beg Rhonda to come to the event with me, and she does. We spend the evening chowing down on fancy cheese and frolicking in the bathroom—a military-style latrine, preserved from when the art space was in fact a home for the armed forces, but also an architectural installation that plays with sound and privacy. It seemed, as I gazed upon a wall of urinals, that life was again and again directing my attention back to bodily fluids.

Two nights later, Quentin comes over straight from his literary debut—at City Lights, no less! He is published in an anthology. Orson is red and teary, having forgotten to take their allergy medicine. The cats, sensing their weakness, climb right up onto them.

"Oh, did you check your email?" Quentin asks. "I sent you my results."

The sperm results! This is almost as exciting as my Clomid coming—which it has not. I want the Clomid to get here, because I want to take it, obviously, but also so I know that I actually gave all my credit card information to an actual, legitimate business and not some sort of scam that charged forty dollars to steal my identity.

I go to my computer and pull up Quentin's results. From what I gather, comparing his results to the standard, he's above average. Quentin! Above average in every way! "That's so great!" I cheer. Even though people say that the dude's sperm needs to be checked for potency, I was never worried about Quentin. He's a virile, healthy twenty-eight-year-old. I know that if there is anything physical preventing this pregnancy from happening, it's on my side. We inseminate me before Orson goes into anaphylactic shock. And again, we begin the wait to see if Quentin's exceptional sperm makes it to my uterus and comes upon an egg eager to make its acquaintance.

THE DAY BEFORE MY FORTY-FIRST BIRTHDAY, I GET THE WEIRDEST PHONE CALL. It's Orson! Orson has NEVER called me on the phone. I answer gingerly, as if it is a serial killer.

". . . . . Hello?"

"Hi."

"Wow, it's your voice," I say.

"I know. Listen, I need you to buzz me into your house, and then go in your kitchen and shut the door. And stay there until I tell you to come out."

"Uh—okay." This is all so mysterious! "Um, bye?"

"Bye," they say, and click away.

I buzz them in, unlock my apartment door, and sit in the kitchen. Or not sit. More like bounce. There is a knock at the door, and I crack it open.

"You can come out now."

In my bedroom is a tree, with fat yellow lemons hanging from it. It's a lemon tree! A miniature Meyer lemon tree! Its leaves are dark and shiny, and I can't believe it's already fruiting. "I don't know if it will live inside a house," Orson cautions, "but if it starts to die, we'll bring it to my mom's. She can save any plant."

I'm touched by the tree. I'd mentioned always wanting one, the fantasy of living in a home naturally scented with the vibrant scent of lemon blossoms, one of my favorite smells. Orson was listening, and what a gift, the gift of something alive. It feels like much more than a plant; it feels like a hopeful omen, or an offering to the powers of nature. I place it in the front room, in front of the wall of windows that look out onto the busy street below. And with that, we head off on my birthday trip to Arcata.

5.

ADVERSITY BONDING

I made sure to pack a bunch of ovulation tests on my Birthday Getaway, though my calculations are a bit of a bummer. It seems I *will* be ovulating this weekend while I'm up in Arcata, land of stoner dudes with dogs on ropes, and while Quentin is back in San Francisco belatedly celebrating *his* birthday by transforming a giant art gallery into a roller-skating rink.

A few days before we left town, I was at home wondering what, in fact, we will do with ourselves once we land in Arcata. I googled "things to do in Arcata" and came upon a redwood zip line adventure. I'm sort of attracted to it—I like going fast, I like the thought of being up in the trees. But I'm also sort of scared of it—I don't like heights and I'm not athletic. I post it on Orson's Facebook, almost as a joke, but they respond immediately: "Yeah, oh my god, I love zip lines, I always wanted to do this!"

And so it goes that we have reservations to zip among the redwood trees early on the morning of my forty-first birthday.

Back before I met Orson, when I had first decided to knock

myself up, my goal was to be pregnant by February eighteenth. A great birthday, by the way. Shared with Yoko Ono, Matt Dillon, Snoop Dogg, Alice Walker, Vince Neil, and Vanna White. In my original plan, if I wasn't with child by my forty-first birthday, I'd call it quits and split for Paris.

I'm glad we got out of town and into the trees on this day. In the forest, anything seems possible. Looking at the redwood trees, which grow in families, little rings of giant, ancient families, life seems like our world's default setting. I *can't* call the pregnancy plan off, not now, not with Orson involved, not with Quentin so dedicated, and not with my new understanding that it can take a long, long time for a person to get pregnant.

Our zip line guy is exactly who you want your zip line guy to be. He's cute and blond and has a fluffy Alaskan sled dog named Stella, who wanders around the grove before hunkering down in a bed of old needles and leaves. He has the vibe of a competent stoner—a stoner who knows not to get stoned before taking a pair of city kids seventy feet up the side of a redwood, but who will likely be hitting the bong at some point this afternoon.

Yes, I did say seventy feet. How will we get all the way up there? It appears we will be climbing. Climbing up the side of a redwood with the help of some rather small, U-shaped steel pegs that have been hammered into the tree in a rather unhelpful pattern. One peg is here, the other way over there, the next is sort of wildly up there, like a rock-climbing wall. I'm baffled, quite worried about how I'm going to do this, but I'm also distracted by having to put on fifty pounds of equipment, including a harness that wraps around me like a giant diaper. Our Hippie explains to us how to clamp on and clamp off, and we run through a practice zip on the ground. This all takes about forty minutes, and by the end, I have psyched myself up for the climb: I'm doing it for OUR BABY!

Parents make all sorts of sacrifices for their children. I've already scaled my coffee back to one single cup per day, so I KNOW what it's like to make a sacrifice. But I'm ready to take it to the next level, seventy feet above the ground. If I'm going to have a baby and be a mom, I can't be scared. Just the physical facts of pregnancy and the terrible possibility of a vaginal birth are enough to make me whimper if I think about it too much; I've got to toughen up! What if I'm called to lift a car off my child, like those adrenaline-powered moms from urban legends?

Also, what about being an awesome role model to our kid—especially to a girl kid? To know that her mom is so tough and fearless would inspire her to be tough and fearless, too. Having a mom who scaled the side of a giant tree would make her feel really safe and protected, wouldn't it? Like her mother actually is a superhero.

Orson goes first, scaling the tree like a monkey. What I see brings back my dread. In this one spot they struggle, stretched to their lanky max. I'm shorter and stumpier. How am I going to shrimp it up that tree?

Once Orson is situated on the top platform, I begin my own scramble. I'm pleased that my hiking boots, thrifted purely for fashion purposes, are seeing some real action. But I'm a little concerned about my jeans. They're tight. They *looked* correct this morning, when I put them on: my townie-style Boston hoodie, these jeans, and my hiking boots. It looked so legitimate, like I was going to shoot an Urban Outfitters catalog posing as a tree-climber. I learned the hard way not to wear tight jeans to meditate at the Zen Center; now it seems another denim lesson is in store, here in the wilds of Arcata.

"You're doing great!" Our Hippie hollers down from the platform, and Orson echoes, "Great job, baby!" I'm breathing pretty hard. I'm relying on Buddhism right now, mindfulness. I can feel muscles I don't use suddenly called into action. I'm doing an okay job staying one peg ahead of my mounting panic, but then I get to this part of the trunk where one peg is right *here* and the next peg is *up there,* and I can't lift my leg high enough to put my boot on it.

"You want to rest?" Our Hippie asks. Orson did it on their way up, it's no big deal. But I'm actually having a bit of a panic attack now. I've got to plow through this. *Focus, focus.* I'm staring straight into the rough, fissured bark of this giant living thing.

"I love you, tree," I tell the tree. I do love the tree. I try to lift my leg higher but can't.

I can always go back down the tree. But would Orson be disappointed in me? They're too understanding to be disappointed, but I wouldn't get to feel how proud they'd be if I kept going. And what about our baby? Did I want our child to think her mom was a wimp, a person who doesn't push herself, doesn't try, succumbs to panic?

I clutch a peg with one hand, and with the other I grab and lift my leg up the side of the tree. I pull myself up and climb onto the next peg. When I hit a lower platform, I slide myself onto it on my belly and just lie there.

"You can take a break, it's totally all right," Our Hippie says cheerfully.

"I'm having a panic attack." It now seems safe to tell them.

"Totally understandable," says Our Hippie, still in his chipper-casual voice. "It's not natural to be so far off the ground." He goes on to tell me about how he went surfing a few days ago and let himself go out farther than he should have and had a panic attack of his own. I lean back against the trunk and try to steady my breathing. Blue sky and golden sunshine come through the cracks of the deep-green canopy. The height doesn't bother me; it was the struggle, my body's feeling of being trapped and incompetent.

I hate—HATE—that I still have to scale another five feet to the final platform, but Orson is up there, and I want to see their face so bad that it fuels the last, complicated stretch, and I'm there.

I feel Orson's pride and am so glad I didn't punk out when things got hard.

"This is just like in *The Bachelor,* when they walked the Bay Bridge together," Orson whispers in my ear. It's our first moment of adversity bonding! My former relationships were nothing but adversity bonding, the adversity being the relationship itself, but Orson and I haven't really had any problems except their PMS that one time, and now this tree.

The zipping is fast and fun and over in like five minutes. It seems ridiculous that you spend so much time prepping and training and climbing the goddamn tree, for just a few minutes of zipping.

"You guys want to go around a few more times?" Our Hippie asks. "This might be a once-in-a-lifetime moment."

"Oh, it is definitely a once-in-a-lifetime moment," I assure him. To zip again means I'd have to climb that five feet between platforms again, and guess what? I never want to do that ever a-fucking-gain.

"I think I'm cool," I say casually.

"Me too," Orson agrees.

Later, we soak in some sort of giant Scandinavian hot tub that looks like the soup pot Elmer Fudd tricks Bugs Bunny into. Those deviant dummies who produce *The Bachelor* really know what they're doing. Forget the thirty-six questions to fall in love. Put two people in a harrowing physical situation and help them survive—*that* is going to form an adversity bond. We let the hot water relax our muscles, sore from effort and anxiety. We hold hands, which grow prunier and prunier as we steep. I feel like I showed Orson that I'm not a quitter, not afraid of hard things, that they could rely on me for the long haul. I am proud of myself, proud of the both of us.

In bed that night, at the Hotel Arcata, I can't sleep for what feels like activity in my womb. It feels hot and jumpy, it feels alive.

All these months studying my body with close eyes, and I was finally becoming attuned to its cycles, its subtle shifts and energies. I'm so glad we inseminated before leaving on this birthday trip. I fall asleep imagining a sperm climbing through my body, up, up, up, till it reaches the top.

6.

MAMA'S TIRED

O n our long drive back to San Francisco, I get a call from
my sister, who is processing the fact that her body is growing a boy.

"Michelle," she says. "What will I do with a *boy?*"

"Just keep an eye on him," say I, the childless, formerly lesbian-
separatist aunt. "Figure out what kind of boy he is."

I'm thinking about my friend Betsy, who just gave birth to a
baby boy. Betsy's partner is genderqueer; assigned female at birth,
they are super manly and identify as a "tweener"—an in-betweener.
Betsy and her tweener also live with a child from the tweener's
previous relationship, a middle schooler already quite learned on
the vast possibilities of gender.

"Actually, we don't know if the baby is really a boy, because
it might grow up and become a girl," the seven-year-old wisely informs everyone about his new sibling.

Folks in my world have separated sex from gender so wholly
that there is no way to comfortably relax into the idea of a baby girl

being like *this,* or a baby boy being like *that.* Which has made my and Orson's name search revolve around What Is a Cute Girl Name That Can Be Easily Converted Into a Cute Boy Name Should Our Child Wind Up Being Transgender and Vice Versa. We're pretty hooked on Theodore for a boy and Theodora for a girl, both having the handy gender-neutral nickname Theo.

Believe me, I would LOVE to name a girl child something hideously looping and feminine, like Isabella or Isadora or Eugenia or Lucretia or Sophia or Antoinette, and I would love to name a boy something eccentrically masculine like Baldwin (after James) or Spencer or Beauford or Maximilian. But—as Orson spent most of their life trying to work with the name Anna—knowing what we know, it may be hard to give our baby a heavily gendered name. I fret over this to the point that I contact Vito and ask him what he thinks. Isn't it inherently problematic to be gendering our baby at all? Obviously we'll always listen to our child's understanding of their self, but shouldn't we make it easier and not introduce gender to them at all?

Vito, who is trans, waves my concerns away. Gender *is* real, it's a thing, and although the project of dismantling the binary will continue, changing culture in ways we can't foresee, the reality is that most people aren't trans, and chances are my kid won't be either. I realize I am living in a deeply queer bubble, where most everyone around me *is* queer and trans. Vito is right. It's enough to be ready for whatever the potential baby expresses, ready to change the name and the pronouns and lead whatever protective charge the parent of a trans or gender-nonconforming child needs to take. I'm so freaking grateful to be queer and to be in this queer community. And I love that whoever my hopeful, eventual baby ends up being, they are going to benefit from this love and wisdom and history as well.

THE NEXT NIGHT, I COME BACK AFTER A DINNER PARTY FUNDRAISER TO FIND A package waiting for me, postmarked India. It's my Clomid! I tear it open as I dash up the stairs, and there is it, foil sheets with little pockets of pills nestled inside. I can't wait to start popping them! Then I remember that I might not have to. My Friday insemination could have possibly gotten me pregnant.

Days later, I'm checking email on my phone while I wait for a flight to Los Angeles to visit Madeline. I find one from Quentin, subject *Immaculate Infection*.

So, it reads. *Remember how my doctor wanted to talk to me about the results of my sperm test? Well, I guess I have a high red blood cell count. And it means I either have a urinary tract infection or gonorrhea. But DON'T WORRY. I CAN'T HAVE gonorrhea. It's just NOT POSSIBLE. It would be the Immaculate Infection! But I'm going to get tested! I don't have insurance anymore, so I have to go to a free clinic. And I'm leaving town, so I'll have to find a clinic while I'm traveling. But DONT WORRY. Because it's NOT EVEN POSSIBLE for me to have gonorrhea.*

I decide to listen to Quentin and not freak out. Surely Quentin, the most wholesome drag queen in the whole world, can't have gonorrhea.

I go on with my travel, and Quentin goes on with his. I receive missives: he's at his parents' house in Upstate New York, sneaking away to the local Planned Parenthood. We were both thrilled with the Afterschool Specialness of Quentin sneaking off to PP like a pregnant teen.

"I didn't even know Planned Parenthood treated men!" I gasped.

"Yeah, gurl." Quentin's next plan is to hit up an STD clinic in Philadelphia. Getting tested at the free clinic seems like a totally natural thing for a queer to do while bumming around the country on their vacay. I'm serious. It really does.

IN LOS ANGELES, I ALLOW MADELINE TO CATCH ME UP ON ALL THE WEIRD POP culture gossip I've somehow missed—even though all I do is ruin my brain with cheap magazines—and that she somehow knows about—even though she is raising a three-year-old and has nary a spare moment for herself.

"You don't know about Kreayshawn?" my sister asks, incredulous. "She lives in Oakland!"

"I don't know what you're talking about!" I insist, and we watch "Gucci Gucci," and then this video of her stoned in some tawdry bedroom with all her creepy gay friends. Not for the first time, I am so grateful there was no internet for me to have posted all the John Waters knock-off "films" me and my friends made while drunk in high school. Meanwhile, Madeline turns her attention toward me and informs me that my boobs are bigger.

"Really?" I ask. I look down at them. "I guess they are," I mumble. They're not *that* much bigger—they're still smaller than my perpetually cheese-bloated belly. But, speaking of bloated, my period is late. In my sister's bathroom, I take another test, imagining how uniquely special it would be to learn I was pregnant here; to get to celebrate with her and hug and hop up and down. But, like the others, it comes back negative.

"I got negative tests for a while with Olivia," Madeline tells me later that afternoon.

"You did?"

My sister nods her head. We are strolling through the L.A. zoo with Olivia. In between gawking at animals, I dash into the bathroom, sure that I keep feeling something in my underwear. Nothing. I cup my breasts. They really are a little bigger. I do a little excited shimmy on the zoo toilet, get up, flush, and return to the animals. Everywhere I look, mamas and babies—a baby gorilla hitching a ride on their mama's back; a joey poking out its head from the coziness of a marsupial pouch. We gawkers point and squeal. "Look at the baby!" Madeline directs Olivia's attention, and I curve my hand around my belly like a prayer to the animal gods.

7.

THE BARNEYS EFFECT

The next day, sometime in the afternoon, I get my period, full-fledged, with cramps and everything.

I'm furious. I am so sick of this shit! This baby-making/baby-failing roller coaster!

I decide to do some internet research. All I ever called was that one fertility clinic, and they didn't even have good Yelp! reviews. Know who does? The big teaching hospital here in San Francisco, where I once had discount dental work performed upon me by a student. I guess you can get fertility work done on you, too. The discounts aren't quite as deep as when you let a newbie rip a tooth out of your head, but online fertility consumers insist that this is the cheapest place with the best reputation. I'm sold.

I make a call, and their financial person calls me right back. I get off the phone feeling like it's less expensive than I thought— maybe not even expensive after all! This is a phenomenon already known to me as the Barneys Effect.

The Barneys Effect: You spend an afternoon drifting around

Barneys in a wonderful altered state of consciousness that is a mélange of anxiety, desire, and fantasy. You take in all the price tags. You read the numbers again and again, until they cease to mean anything. They're just some sort of code. Some numbers are higher, and some are lower. Slowly—slowly—the lower numbers start to feel . . . low. One thousand dollars is a lot less expensive than ten thousand dollars. After looking at Rodarte ball gowns, a Phillip Lim shift seems to be AN ACTUAL STEAL. It's not. It's like eight hundred dollars. That's expensive. You are a moron. But you know what? It feels good to be a moron. Sort of drifting through an enchanted forest of a fantasy life feeling your brain become addled as items that cost as much as your actual rent begin to seem totally reasonable.

At this point, you should have a moment of clarity and get your ass out of Barneys *now*. Run, don't walk, to the sale rack at Urban Outfitters, where items cap off at $39.99. Barneys has made the sale rack at Urban Outfitters look like a tag sale at a small-town church in rural New England. YOU CAN HAVE ANYTHING YOU WANT. You can leave with five new items that cost you, total, less than a pair of socks at Barneys.

I think the Barneys Effect is coming into play now, as I shop for fertility help. Recognizing that the large sums of money owed at the teaching hospital are smaller than the large sums of money required at the fertility clinics, I suddenly feel like I'm at the sale rack at Urban Outfitters and can have ANY FERTILITY PROCEDURE I WANT.

I make an appointment with a fertility specialist and hang up the phone. When I come back into my body I find myself on the verge of tears. So much for the Barneys Effect! Spending money terrifies me. And I don't think it matters how much money I'll ever have or ever won't have, because it's not rational. I remember reading some article in a gossip rag about how Madonna—surely a millionaire many times over—is actually very anxious about spending money. The tone of the article suggested we should be outraged by this decadent person who has become so rich, she has lost all touch with reality, but I just felt bad for her, the girl who grew up motherless in Detroit. You don't have to be poor to lose track of reality when it comes to money.

But this investment, I feel, has to be worth it, and so I make the appointment for the end of the month. What will I do between now and then? How about some internet research on how Clomid *doesn't really work on women over the age of thirty-five*. You're kidding! Who the fuck even needs Clomid if *not* women over the age of thirty-five! Or are all women just super infertile now from pesticides and BPA in our canned foods and whatever endocrine disrupters are leaching from our bottled water or just the air itself?

I shift gears, making an appointment with a gynecologist and locating a sensible lesbian GP. Orson has put me on their health insurance. They didn't make a big deal about it—it almost felt like an act of charity, like how could someone stand by and watch a person try to get pregnant in the broken arms of the free-clinic system? I followed their lead, not making a big deal about it either. I thought about the time, many years ago, when I had Kaiser through a job and lent Tali my HMO card to get her back looked at. Queers help each other out. But I felt that, beneath the surface, in Orson's introverted way, they were taking care of me.

I won't say that I've never had health insurance as an adult, because it's not true. In 1993 I worked for one year at a housing nonprofit that gave me insurance. And in 2009 I was briefly employed by a prestigious college and had Kaiser. But in the twenty-three years of my adulthood, I've spent twenty-one of them uninsured. Suddenly having health insurance is so unreal that it takes me a month to get it together. I call my new insurer to see if they offer any kind of fertility benefits.

"You mean *infertility* benefits?" the lady on the line corrects me. I guess so. But I don't *know* that I'm infertile—I'm trying to find out! Regardless, my new health insurance does not cover it. Not many insurance agencies do. I feel a little disappointed but snap out of it quickly. At least I have proper health insurance and can stop struggling within the complicated free-clinic system.

That rainy night, my insemination team meets up at my house. Rhonda, who has had enough of Bay Area housing misery and moved to Los Angeles, is in town. Quentin—officially STD free!—shows up in a tizzy. There's much to discuss. He got into grad school! It's very exciting, in theory. The same denial mechanism that has blocked me from comprehending that Rhonda has moved to Los Angeles disconnects my brain when I attempt to calculate how much time that leaves us with Quentin and his sperm. I've got to amp up my body's fertility somehow if I'm going to get pregnant before Quentin moves on with the rest of his life. I remember the initial deal I'd made with myself, or with the Universe: I'd try to get pregnant, and if it didn't work, shrug it off and go to Paris. Now that I was in the groove of it all—the rise and fall of hope, the growing involvement of Orson, the unexpected emotional investment—how was I to know if it "didn't work"? How many tries were enough? Was Quentin's imminent departure a sign, or was I to chase him out to the coastal university where he'd be studying? It wasn't *that* far . . .

Quentin is dressed as Miss Super Extra Deluxe Pandemonium. She is wearing a denim onesie, fake nails decorated with glittered starbursts, hot pink lips, false eyelashes that look like giant, glamorous spiders, open-toe leopard stilettos, a pink scarf knotted around her neck, and a pink pleather belt cinched around her waist. She goes into the kitchen, removes two of the fake nails, and gets to work.

As I lie in bed, letting Quentin's sperm sashay up my cervix, I muse on how hard it will be not getting inseminated next month. I'll be traveling all month with my performance tour, Sister Spit. Orson is coming to visit me two weeks into the tour—what if I happen to be ovulating then? Could they bring the sperm on the plane? Could they get it through security?

"You'd have to be bold," Rhonda advises sternly. Everyone Googles "sperm on planes" while I lie on my back. We reach a consensus that it's not a very good plan.

I'M ON A BUS HEADED TO THE MARINA, WHERE MY NEW GYNECOLOGIST IS. THIS is my first appointment not at a free clinic in years, and I'm psyched! The insurance card in my wallet feels like a toy. I'm going to get SO HEALTHY! Except, when I get to the front desk, the young lady informs me that my new gynecologist is not there and my appointment has been canceled. "Didn't you get our message?" she asks. "We called you."

"I didn't get the message," I tell the receptionist, hyperventilating. I'm breaking out in a sweat, an instant mess. My years in the public health system have possibly left me with a bit of PTSD, quick to go off the rails when something goes awry. In the public health system it can take *forever* to see a doctor. If anything gets canceled—which it frequently does—you are left back at square one, delayed for weeks or months. I'm ready to fight for my right to be seen today, even though it's my own fault this happened, because like an alcoholic hitting bottom, I have just stopped answering my telephone.

But guess what? I'm not at the free clinic. I have been elevated to the elite class of the insured. And it *is* a class. Thanks to my particular partner and their particular good job, I'm in. The receptionist has barely clocked the haywire shift in my demeanor. She's too busy trying to help me.

"Dr. Becky can see you instead," she tells me sweetly, and urges me toward the frosted-glass waiting room with its racks of magazines. I take a seat and collect myself. It's amazing how, though I really think of myself as pretty fucking together, I am pretty quick to come apart. The people here want to help me. Amazing! Not that free clinic workers don't want to help, too—they probably want to help more than anyone. But days working with demographics experiencing intense, chronic physical and mental challenges, being overworked and underpaid, having funding so unstable that patients do burlesque shows and bake sales to keep you in business—it just creates a different environment. In comparison, this office is positively serene.

Dr. Becky calls me into her office, which has a great wooden desk and is filled with optimism. Dr. Becky is kind of hot. She's wearing a tight black dress, short, with a cutaway at her sternum. It would almost be inappropriate except she's wearing a tight, long-sleeved shirt beneath it, and leggings and leather boots. She's also wearing the silver bean necklace from Tiffany that Anne Hathaway's character wears in *The Devil Wears Prada,* which I know all about, because it has been my sister's signature piece of jewelry for years. I feel like this is an omen of the highest degree.

Dr. Becky asks me all the questions doctors ask you, including what medications I am currently on. "Generic Celexa," I tell her. "And Clomid that I bought off the internet." I wait to be scolded, but Dr. Becky is fascinated and a bit amused. I think she might admire my pluck!

"Where did it come from?" she asks. "Mexico?"

"India," I report. I explain my pregnancy attempts.

"That is so great that you have a known donor helping you out!" She smiles. Is this bougie doctors' office actually as nonjudgmental as my queer free clinic? This is too good to be true!

We leave her spacious office and move into an exam room that has the latest *Vogue* in the magazine rack. Dr. Becky examines my breasts and compliments my tattoos. "'Prudence Never Pays,'" she says, reading some text around a tattooed heart.

"It's from a Smiths song," I explain, confident that Dr. Becky will know who the Smiths are. "I got it in Manchester, England. Where they're from."

"I was more into the Dickies," she says. "But I think I'm a little older than you."

Dr. Becky is PUNK! What is this alternative world I have rabbit-holed into? I actually feel cared for, like Dr. Becky and her people *want* to help me, not like a burden to be shuffled out quickly so as to quickly shuffle in the next burden. I realize that this PTSD has been a big part of my aversion to going to a fertility doctor. It didn't occur to me that I could have a positive health care experience.

As I'm having this deep revelation that my entire life is a process of ferreting out my PTSD and then healing it, Dr. Becky has her hand up my snatch. She presses down on my abdomen with her free hand. "Are you sure you're not pregnant?" she asks. "Your uterus is enlarged."

My heart stops. WHAT? Dr. Becky is an ob-gyn. Surely she would not whimsically suggest that I *could* be pregnant if that wasn't a serious possibility.

"When did you last test?" she asks.

"I got my period, and I stopped," I told her.

"Some women mistake their implantation bleeding for their period," she says. "You should test again. I'd say you could be at six weeks, but you also might have a tilted cervix, so I'm not getting the best read on it."

I want to kill Dr. Becky for reviving my dashed hopes, but I love her too much to hate her.

"I don't do OB anymore," Dr. Becky tells me, "but I'll be your GYN wench until you're pregnant, and then I'll hook you up with someone really great." As she says this I understand that Dr. Becky fully assumes that I will, at some point, be pregnant. And she's a *professional,* an expert on eggs and uteruses (uteri?) and fallopian tubes and babies. If she believes I can get pregnant, it seems only logical that I believe it, too.

8.

RIDDLED WITH FIBROIDS

This will be our last insemination for forever!" Quentin says sadly, days before I embark on my spoken word tour. Then, remembering why we're all there, he corrects himself: "Oh! Well, I mean, I hope it's the last one truly forever!" Quentin is in drag again, Arts Admin Drag: satin pants, a bronze blouse, and a wrap, all in autumnal tones. His hair is long and curly, and he's wearing very intellectual-looking eyeglasses. I totally feel like she's going to review my grant application and give me some stern but loving feedback.

I bust out a bottle of Martinelli's sparkling cider and Quentin, Rhonda, Orson, and I raise our glasses for a toast. We've all come together over these months to take a tremendous, intimate risk together. Rhonda has stared down my vagina. Quentin has engaged in one of the most personal of acts, in my kitchen, my cats clawing at the door. Orson has held a bowl of sperm and globbed it up into a syringe. It all could have been horribly awkward, and while it may have been *occasionally* awkward, it was never horrible. I understand why Quentin is feeling sentimental about the break we'll be having. Though the main objective has been to get me pregnant, what we created was a strange, personal gathering where we all grew closer. Like a book club. Sperm Club.

BEFORE I LEAVE FOR TOUR, I HAVE A VISIT WITH THE FERTILITY CLINIC AT THE teaching hospital.

My name is called, and I am led to my doctor, Dr. Waller, by a person who appears to be a big dyke, with short, buzzed hair and short fingernails. If there is in fact a lesbian gene, I think Jan is carrying it. I can't believe my good fortune!

In Dr. Waller's room, Jan goes through my intake form with me. It feels sort of bad to reflect on these things. No, I don't know if my birth father is alive or dead; last I heard, he was alive, but that was some years ago, and he'd told me he was having heart problems, and then his phone got disconnected, and who knows. I think his brothers are all alcoholics and one had cirrhosis. I don't know anything about my paternal grandmother. Ugh. Do I even want to pass on these genes?

I tell Jan about what we've been doing, the inseminations, and I tell her about Orson. "Queer families are so great," she says knowingly. "You have so many more options." She leads me into the exam room for my ultrasound with Dr. Waller.

Dr. Waller has little spectacles and a chipper, somewhat humorous manner. It would be unfair to compare anyone to Dr. Becky, whom I am in love with, but on the scale of doctor warmth, he's actually pretty up there. I'm given a moment of privacy to take off my pants and underwear and hop up on the exam table, a paper sheet across my thighs.

I've had an ultrasound before, and they slid an object across my greased-up belly. That's what I was expecting. I was not expecting an instrument that looks like a big vibrator to be stuck up my va-

gina. Well, I think, at least Jan is a lesbian. At least I am being vaginally probed by someone who likely has years of experience, both
professional and otherwise. And it is true that Jan is a way more
skillful wand-wielder than Dr. Waller. When the doctor takes over,
the wand becomes a joystick, and I, a video game. He twists and
jerks the thing around like he's trying to blow up asteroids.

"Wow," Dr. Waller says. Game over? "You are *riddled* with fibroids. Did you know that?"

Did I know that I was *riddled* with fibroids? "No," I say.

The doctor finds this hard to believe.

"You're not in pain? No heavy periods, painful periods?"

"Nnnnnno," I say.

"I mean, one is about seven centimeters," Dr. Waller elaborates.
"It totally obscures your right ovary, I'm getting no picture of the
eggs there. But your left ovary has a less-than-average egg count."

"Less than average?" I repeat. I'm getting a lot of information at
once, all with an alien probe lodged up my snatch. "Like, less than
the average woman my age has?"

"Yeah," Dr. Waller confirms. "And, at your age, sixty to eighty
percent of the eggs you do have aren't viable anyway."

Well, this certainly doesn't sound like good news. Sixty to eighty
percent of my eggs are busted, and I have fewer eggs than the average forty-one-year-old. And I'm riddled with fibroids.

Jan and Dr. Waller leave me to collect my dignity and my
clothes. This is why Dr. Becky thought I could be six weeks pregnant. It wasn't a fetus up there, it was—what the fuck are fibroids,
anyway? Hair and teeth? My little fuzzy monster baby?

Back in Dr. Waller's office, conversation turns to Orson. How
old is Orson? Orson is thirty-two. This pleases Dr. Waller greatly.
"Their eggs are *infinitely* healthier than yours," he tells me.

"Really?"

"*Infinitely.*"

I believe he means for me to find relief in this statement, but instead I'm on the verge of tears. The reality of all those sweet insemination gatherings hits me. With my low egg count and advanced age and fibroid-riddled uterus, I was never going to get pregnant. I wasted everyone's time. I pledge that I am *not* going to cry in front of queer Jan and the doctor. I do some breathing tricks and try to think of neutral things, like fog or hamburgers. Shrubbery. Telephone poles. Flip-flops.

Back in the lobby, I send Orson a darkly humorous text that surely reads as a cry for help: *My eggs are busted*, I type. *You're up.* They call immediately, and I sit in a plush chair by the elevator that is clearly the post-appointment emotional lady's crying chair, replete with a box of Kleenex. Still, I refuse to cry. I tell Orson briefly what I've learned. I can feel them worry for me through the phone, but there's nothing to be done. They're at work, and I've decided to blow off my own workday and just wander aimlessly in a daze until I can see them later on.

I find a breakfast place that not only has an amazing, swanky atmosphere, maple sugar bacon, and crazy pancakes; it has a whole table piled with magazines you can read while you eat. One of the premiere pleasures of life is sitting alone in a restaurant, eating, and reading a magazine. I grab a bunch and settle down with a bottomless cup of coffee. I plan to get massively wired. It no longer matters how much caffeine I consume.

After my breakfast, I wander in the fog toward a Goodwill, and spend a couple hours drifting around the shop in a fugue state, selecting items and then abandoning them. I wind up with a J.Crew raincoat, as it has started to rain. Every now and then something surges inside me, and I think, that's a feeling. But then it goes away. I worry I'm not feeling my feelings enough. Should I try to make myself cry or something? The tears that felt close in the doctor's office now feel caught in my throat. I'm breathing around them.

I think about how, if I were crying, I'd be trying to get myself collected, and now here I am collected, trying to make myself cry, and that there isn't any proper way to deal with this stupid moment except allowing myself whatever treat, food, coffee, and second-hand clothing items I want. So that's my plan.

I'd wondered how I'd know when it was time to stop trying. It seems like this should be it, medical confirmation that my eggs are both scarce and subpar. But I guess the past months have shifted my priority. Paris felt like as good a consolation as the pair of Melissa jelly flip-flops I find at the Goodwill. I realize, as I pay for them at the counter, that I don't really want them so much as I *want* to want them. I want back that irreverent ambivalence I had at the start of the baby project, but too much has happened. I've invested too much. I've made the mistake I'd always guarded against making: wanting something I really can't have.

9.

BUTCH BABY RANCH

We have to get you pregnant," I say to Orson that night. Orson looks alarmed. No, that's not right. It's more that a look of sheer terror moves across their face and freezes there. "Now?" they exclaim. "I'm not ready!"

Before meeting me, Orson assumed that someday they would have to figure out how to give birth—though the idea horrified them—because the thought of finding a femme to have their baby struck them as sort of crude. But now that they *have* unwittingly found a femme to have their baby, the thought of getting their half-man, half-woman body/mind/spirit pregnant is a bit unbearable.

"I understand," says my sister, when I tell her about Orson's reluctance to get knocked up. "Being pregnant is *so miserable,* even if you don't have body issues. I can't imagine how awful it would be for Orson."

I think of Orson going to work, where they lead and direct more or less as a guy. They wear tailored menswear. They're regarded as male. They *are* male. They're a male female. To have their belly and tits suddenly surge out of control, to walk through the world like that, is too much for them.

"I'd have to go to a farm or something," they say, truly trying to problem-solve an unsolvable problem. I imagine us retiring to a yurt in the woods for nine months, where I would minister to my pregnant boyfriend, giving massages and making stews with herbs I forage from the forest.

"Butch baby ranch!" my friend Gertrude enthuses over the telephone. Her butch girlfriend also might be the bearer of their eventual baby and is having similar body issues. The problem has sparked Gertrude's can-do, entrepreneurial spirit—she'll open a ranch, a Butch Baby Ranch, sort of like those places in Nevada where women used to go for divorces in the fifties, only, at the ranch, butch people whose bodies are betraying them with the miracle of life can hide out and butch bond over their bulging butch bellies.

That this is actually a fantastic idea is confirmed by how excited my brother-in-law, a reality television producer, gets about it. It would make a really great show! I get totally excited, too. I know it's trashy, but I'd just love to be on a reality show! I buzz around a bit high from the idea until I realize a reality show about Butch Baby Ranch would sort of defeat the purpose. The menfolk would be showing up to hide from the public, not to be broadcast to millions. Oh well.

Orson thinks that, whatever else happens, I need to get those fibroids removed. The thought doesn't totally stress me out. I know enough people who've had the procedure that it feels pretty common, and now that I have health insurance, it doesn't seem like a financial apocalypse. Orson also is slow to give up on the possibility of me going forward with some sort of treatment, like an IUI.

"The odds are so low," I explain, "and the cost is so high, we'd be better off going on a gambling spree and hiring a surrogate with our winnings." Truly, we could find a way through the financial mess of it if there was more of a guarantee of a baby on the other end, but it seems like only a fool or a really, really rich person would take this route.

"Let's just wait, and think on it," Orson says. But we can't think on anything for too long where my low-end eggs are concerned. Every moment we deliberate, another one spoils. We think on me going forward, against the odds. We think on Orson sucking it up and getting knocked up and being put through woman-body hell for most of a year. We think of adoption, as do many others. We may not relate to the baby-mad straight ladies who post about their yearnings on the internet, but we now have far more in common with them than I ever thought we would. I feel paralyzed with how many routes are seemingly available to us, yet how impossible they all feel at the moment.

"I'm looking into Polish adoption for you," my sister tells me, which is very cute. Lots of people keep talking to me about adoption, and I know it's plausible, and something we might choose in order to expand our theoretical brood. I'm totally open to it, too—it's just not my first choice. My first choice would be having the whole experience of pregnancy, which I have a gut feeling I'd enjoy, despite how grueling it can be. I crave it in a weird, mysterious manner. How can you crave something you've never known? It is so strange.

A lot of folks have reminded me that there are a lot of unwanted children in the world, which does nothing to spur me toward adoption but only makes me feel bad, like my desire to have a baby is wrong and a correct desire would be a more selfless impulse to save a child in need. But for me, these are two different desires. My sadness at the thought of unwanted children lives in the same part of my mind that feels sadness at the homeless men I see sprawled out and beat up on the curbs in my city, or the thoughts of people being murdered in Syria, or raped women forced by law to carry their unwanted child to term. It is stashed with all the other heaps of injustices, both general and specific, and feels very, very different from this desire to walk around with something alive inside my body for nine months.

Nonetheless, I sit down with a deck of tarot cards. I pick three cards on adopting a child. The cards are not great. Okay. I pick three more cards, on Orson having our baby. Again, gloomy or uninspiring cards pop up. I shuffle again, asking the deck if I am supposed to go forward with IUIs or IVF with Dr. Waller. Three more lousy cards come out.

You'd think that maybe this means I'm not supposed to have a baby at all, but the tarot reading I did at the very start of this whole thing said otherwise. I got glowing, lovely, radiant cards that said YES. Maybe, then, you'd think that tarot cards are a bunch of bullshit and I'm a moron for trusting such important life decisions to them, but I've been reading tarot for too long—twenty-six years—to feel that way. Regardless, I'm stumped. And I figure that's just how I'm supposed to be right now. Stumped, stymied, in limbo. At least I'm about to leave on tour and won't be able to do anything for a month anyway. I split town without telling Quentin and Rhonda what I've learned about my body.

10.

ALL I WANNA TO DO
IS MAKE LOVE TO YOU

Being on tour and away from my life could have been a nice break from my pregnancy quest, except that I'd decided to read about it at our shows. It's the only writing that feels fresh and interesting to me, so I perform it every night, little memoiresque narratives about what I've been doing with my life. I camp it up, stressing the absurdity of it all, and the audience's laughter feels like a tiny reward for all that has happened. I'm so glad I'm a writer. Every experience, no matter how futile-seeming, can always be redeemed later, in a story. Every night I both read and host the variety-style show, cashing in on my own redemption via audience applause, and in turn clapping for the other writers, all of whom use the roller coaster of randomness that is life as the inspiration for the personal stories they share. They are, truly, my heroes.

However, after every performance, someone inevitably comes up and asks me if I'm pregnant. I knew this would happen and have accepted it. I'm used to being asked personal questions after a show—that's what you get when you read about your personal life on a stage in front of a hundred people, making jokes about it and seeming infinitely comfortable with the world knowing your business. People come up to you later and ask you about fisting, or your difficult relationship with your parents, or how your ex feels about what you just wrote. I always hope it won't happen, because, in spite of everything, I actually don't like talking about my personal life with strangers. I really don't. There is a major disconnect in being able to write about my private shames, perform them in the magical and protected-feeling space of a stage, and then have to discuss it with people you don't know.

I don't expect anyone to get this, or even be sympathetic toward it. I get that I can't have it both ways. Which is why I politely chirp, "No, not yet!" when asked about the baby after the show. I'm used to being slightly out of my body after hosting an hour-and-a-half show. I figured the weird autopilot would coast me through the discomfort, and it mostly does. Mostly.

After Erin Markey, an artist who each night enacts a play based on her relationship with her mother, dreams of the Heart song "All I Wanna Do Is Make Love to You," we are forced to listen to it on repeat for a few hundred miles. The culture inside this van, where a bunch of weirdo artists are cohabiting for thirty days, is so surreal that this is more or less acceptable. Also, the rigors of living on the road are real, and we all try to be very accommodating of one another's needs. And Erin needs to listen to this song. A lot.

Eventually, after a heavy dissection and analysis of the song's lyrics, Erin proclaims that the "one little thing" the narrator's lover can give her, that her husband can't give her, is not an orgasm. It's a BABY!

"Are you sure she doesn't mean an orgasm?" I challenge.

"No!" Erin exclaims. "'Imagine his surprise, when he saw his own eyes.'"

"Hmmmm . . ."

"And she says, 'Don't try to find me, please don't you dare,' because she doesn't want him to find the kid!" Erin continues, high on cracking this mystery after a couple hours of heavy rotation.

"Well, her partner is shooting blanks," chimes Cassie J. Sneider, a writer who has been reading each night about her family getting attacked by monkeys at an amusement park.

"That's what I think, too!" Erin exclaims. "It's like the most feminist *and* most misogynist song of all time."

We give it another listen. I suddenly feel camaraderie with the narrator and the extreme efforts she makes to get herself knocked up.

"You guys don't understand," I say, knowingly nodding my head to the music. "Baby fever is *real.*"

ME AND ORSON HAVE A PACT: NO MORE THAN TWO WEEKS CAN GO BY WITHOUT us seeing each other. I've been touring regularly since the nineties, and I know all too well what distance can do to a relationship. Every single relationship I've been in has collapsed after a tour. Sometimes it was my fault, like back in the nineties when I was such a wild alcoholic and would get carried away on the road, partying every night in a different city. I would just *forget* that I was in a committed relationship. On a couple occasions, I went ahead and started whole new relationships inside the strange bubble of the van, which after a week or so feels like the only life you have ever known. I have no concerns of anything like that happening ever again. I believe Orson's heart and mine are true. But mostly I'm just a little superstitious.

We make a plan for them to come and meet me in the Midwest and travel around with the group. I'm psyched that they will get to experience the insanity of a performance tour—the shows, the van, the chaos of flying on airplanes—with me. After the shows, we split off from the group and our necessarily budget hotels, spending the night someplace fancy all by ourselves. We feel very away from our regular lives in San Francisco, caught up in the frenzied rhythms of tour, waking up in Chicago in the morning, running around a Colorado college campus and grabbing dinner from vending machines in the student union that evening.

After the performance, we're walking through downtown Denver when we pass a girl who looks about fifteen years old. She has a sulky face and is leaning against a brick wall, smoking a ciga-rette. She looks to be about eight months pregnant.

We are gripped with the crazed impulse to turn around and beg the girl for her baby. It seems to strike us both at once—the smoke from her cigarette wafts into our faces, we look toward her, take in her belly, her youthful demeanor—and we glance back at each other, eyes wide. Her brazen cigarette smoking on a busy street seems an obvious cry for help.

"Do we ask that girl for her baby?" I say, feeling totally insane, and yet. Such things happen, do they not? It's the stuff of Lifetime movies. Or, at least, the stuff of novels.

"We can't," Orson says. "It's— No. We can't."

"Right." I nod.

"But—oh my god. I mean—should we?"

We walk for a couple blocks reeling from how this strong impulse has knocked us off-kilter. It's a maniacal thing to do. We can't bum a baby off a smoking teenager. Right? We're out of our minds. Slowly, our quick obsession with this baby and its mother—herself a kid in obvious need of some parents—turns into an obsession with our obsession. Look at what has happened to us. We can't let this go. Even at rest, some part of our minds is at work, problem-solving, gears cranking, figuring out how to get us a goddamned baby. One thing was for sure—it wasn't going to happen that night, there, in Denver, Colorado. We go back to our hotel room.

11.

DON'T LOOK BACK

Home from tour, I make an appointment with Dr. Becky in the Marina to talk to her about my fibroids.

"I love to do surgery," Dr. Becky tells me happily in the exam room. Dr. Becky describes the robot-assisted laparoscopic surgery that will remove the fibroids I'm "riddled" with. I imagine a colony of mushrooms have popped up inside me. I hate mushrooms.

The procedure will be done via little slits made in my abdomen. "You'll have scars," she warns me, but that doesn't bother me too much. I also tell her about the news I got from Dr. Waller, that I'll never get pregnant on my own and that my ovaries are impoverished. The fertility clinic and its high-priced poking and prodding beckons.

"Make up your mind and don't look back," Dr. Becky advises. The words ring in my head. *Make up your mind and don't look back.*

At home, I pick another tarot card about my conundrum. The

Devil. A beer-bellied, winged Beelzebub perches on a block of stone; chained to it are some naked, enslaved humans. That's me. The fertility clinic feels larger than me, like it has some sort of control over my life. I'm helplessly floundering at its feet.

I fumble with the tarot cards, wishing there was something else I could ask the deck. I've drawn cards about adoption, IUI, and Orson carrying our baby, and they were all meh, or worse. Suddenly, a whole new option occurs me: What about fertilizing one of Orson's "infinitely healthier" eggs—and then *I* carry it? Unlike the horror that grips Orson when they imagine their own egg being fertilized within them, the thought of transferring one of their youthful eggs into *me* fills them with purpose and excitement. I decide to pull some cards on it.

As I shuffle the deck, I ponder the pros and cons. Pros: a baby. I get to experience being pregnant. With Orson's egg in play, we both get to be more physically involved. As much as we don't really care about passing on our genes and whatnot, it *is* cute that the baby would look like Orson. The baby would have Orson's DNA blueprint, built with materials from my own body. A real collaboration. Cons: it's the most expensive option. That's really the only con I can think of.

I pick three cards off the top of the deck. Art, Virtue, Works. In the Crowley deck I'm reading with, the Art card is a marriage card. It's about two people creating something together. It's a beautiful, strong card.

The Virtue card, which is three of wands, is always read as a *yes* card to me. I tell people that it's like the Universe patting you on the back and saying, *Good job, you're on the right track.* It's the Sun in Aries, maybe a little headstrong but totally positive. One mysterious read on it says, "Out of the two comes three."

The final card is three disks, Mars in Capricorn, Works. Your Mars is your engine, your ambition; to have it in Capricorn means you have a goal, something to achieve, something you are pledged to strive toward. Since Capricorns were built to win it guarantees success—if you work for it. Not only is this the best reading of the bunch, it's just a really great reading.

Things have progressed with Orson, and the next month, they (and Rodney) are going to move into my apartment. The cats will go to a brilliant seventeen-year-old queer writer I'm mentoring. I'm really enjoying our final month in Orson's miniature one-bedroom, where we first had sex and first said I love you.

I tell Orson that I made the appointment for them to see Dr. Waller, and they squeal with excitement and nerves. We make out in the waning sunlight, and in between kisses I prep them on what to expect.

"He's going to take this—wand," I warn them, "and put it up your hooch." Orson makes a terrible face. "He's going to go like this with it," I say, and mime like I am ransacking their inner space with a light saber. "It's like he's playing a video game. He's going to get it up there and clear a screen of Pac-Man." Orson gulps.

We lay together in Orson's bed, talking about sperm. After everything I've put Quentin through, I can't bring myself to ask him to join us on this next round. Plus, Orson is made nervous by the thought of our child's donor being around us. What if some unknown feelings erupt? What if there is drama, problems? But Orson can't get fully comfortable with the idea of sperm banks either.

"Do sperm banks let donors donate again and again?" Orson wonders. They don't like the thought of our kid having unknown siblings out there. I happen to find the idea of learning that you've got siblings in the world sort of mysterious and thrilling, but Orson and I are different. Wild expanses of uncharted territory invigorate me: secrets to decode, mysteries to unravel. Orson tends toward safety, stability, organization. No surprise family member popping out at us like a jack-in-the-box for them. After all, both of us knew, from our own experience, how toxic family can be. We'd done so much to heal from our own family dynamics; what if we were inviting someone else's messed-up relations into our own protected space?

"I wish they didn't get paid for it," they continue. "We have to make sure the kid can meet the guy when they're older."

"Yeah," I agree.

"That will be scary for us," they say.

My mind flashes to the movie *The Kids Are All Right*. "It won't be so bad," I tell them. "Maybe one of us will get to have sex with Mark Ruffalo."

In the morning, I ring up the fertility clinic and explain to Nancy, our case manager, the new plan: I will carry Orson's fine, young egg. Nancy begins routing our path into this scenario, and mentions that we'll have to have a psych consult. A psych consult! Do all couples have to undergo psych consults, or just queer ones? I'm so *ready* to be gaybashed in this process! I can't tell if my vigilance is warranted or if I'm totally damaged and easily triggered or what. Nancy assures me that psych consults are required for all "*fertilized embryo transfers*," which is what we're doing. In their computer, I am now the "patient" and Orson is the "donor."

When I first started investigating fertility clinics, I had presumed that most people seeking these services would be queer—lesbian couples, primarily. It's been a shock to see how heterosexual the system is, so much so that the clinic's computer system isn't capable of listing me and Orson as a couple. It's more like Orson is a young surrogate whom I'm buying an egg off, so that me and my husband can have a kid. It's creepy and annoying. Even though I'm seeing that lesbos aren't the majority clients here, there still has had to be enough of us to make accommodating us worthwhile. Right? Or enough of them getting annoyed that there'd be some complaining? But here I am, seething in silence. Because the whole effort is intimidating and emotionally exhausting, and it's hard to get it up for a freedom fight in the midst of it. I engage in some cost-benefit analysis, a familiar enough equation to sort. What will leave me in a better mental state at the end: trying to educate a worker who is likely exhausted at her job and not super inclined to take on the task of changing the systemic queerphobia inherent in their process, or taking a breath, letting it go, and moving on? I take a breath. I let it go. I move on.

12.

FEET IN THE FEETY HOLDERS

It is the start of a very big week for me and Orson. They are preparing to have their eggs evaluated, and I am prepping to have my fibroids removed via a robot and Dr. Becky. She says I'll be out of commission for two weeks, but I find it hard to believe that my body won't just snap back into perfection after about three or four days. That's *my* plan, at least. There's no time to waste, as I'm also prepping for Orson and Rodney to move in. This means getting rid of a lot of things—selling clothes, getting rid of my lovely antique French bed, giving my cat-scratched leather chairs away. I leave stacks of plates and dishes on the free pile at the foot of my stairs. A neighbor takes my toaster oven, then returns it. I move my dining room table into my bedroom, which will become a living room featuring Orson's wide-screen TV. Orson is a television watcher. My relationship to TV is similar to my relationship to cooking: I like to do it with another person. Left on my own, I'll read books and eat crackers. But soon I'll have cable! And we're going to buy an *adult* couch, one that will take us through the long haul.

In addition to prepping for surgery, shopping for adult furniture, purging half of my belongings, and getting ready for Orson's own appointment at the fertility clinic, we learn we have fleas. FLEAS. A plague of them, biblical style.

How can this be? I've been living with the cats for nearly a year, and never have I seen a flea! I text the queer teen who now has them: *Hey, um, do Harry and Mancha have fleas?*

Nope, she replies.

I know I have fleas because I've been bringing Rodney over to my house each afternoon to get him used to his new home, and every night he returns to Orson with a bellyful of bugs.

I understand that asshole fleas can lay dormant in your home for a millennium, especially in a hardwood-floor home like mine. I just don't understand why they never attacked the cats. Do some fleas prefer dogs to cats? The process to rid Rodney of them is disgusting, but if, Goddexx willing, we are to someday be with child, there are many disgusting processes we'll have to bravely face: poopy butts, spontaneous vomit, head lice. I accept the challenge as I do all challenges these days, as an undertaking that is just prepping me to be a better mom.

I HAVE A PRE-OP APPOINTMENT WITH DR. BECKY, WHO ARRIVES FRESH FROM A surgery. Her hair is disheveled, no doubt from a recent surgical cap, and the rings that normally gleam on her fingers today sway on a chain around her neck. She also has a different energy, a heightened vibe. It might just be from running around, but I wonder if doing surgeries are a sort of high for Dr. Becky. She had expressed her love of the work; perhaps it gives her dopamine, the way getting lost in writing, when it's going well, can leave me buzzed on my own brain chemistry.

Lying back on the exam bed, I lift my shirt so the doctor can poke me in all the spots I'll be cut.

"You'll have a second bellybutton," she says lightly, pressing gently on my tummy about half an inch above my innie. Then she touches the right side of my abdomen and makes a regretful face. "This scar will be the painful one," she tells me. "It's where the robot will enter to chew the fibroids."

Chew the fibroids. Ew. I can't wait to tell this eventual child of mine all the gnarly shit I had to do to bring them into the world.

———

A DAY LATER, I'M IN THE WAITING ROOM AT THE FERTILITY CLINIC, HUDDLED INTO Orson on a small couch, talking shit while they shush me. "I mean, 'No Children'?" I read the sign on the clinic wall, asking patients to leave other children at home. "Ladies need to toughen up. You can't zone the world to protect you from getting triggered."

"Shhh!" Orson hushes my rant.

"Are you ready for Dr. Waller to play pinball with your vagina?" I ask. They look at me askance. "I mean Atari! Are you ready for him to play Atari with your vagina? I'm sorry, my mistake." I crack up into their shoulder.

"No laughing!" Orson scolds me. Recently, Orson confessed that even though they would *never* want me to do *anything different,* because they want me to be *myself,* they do wish that I would put my dinner napkin on my lap, and wait till all the other diners' food arrives before eating at a restaurant. I also had a bad habit of spitting out my gum on the street until Orson educated me on the error of my ways. I am not as classy as Orson, and my fertility clinic guffaws, plus my dining habits, confirm this.

While I judge the women who can't handle the sight of someone else's child, Orson is judging all the men who are conspicuously absent. Why aren't they here with their Wimmin, supporting them and holding their hands? I remind them that *they* hadn't come with *me* when I got my vag wanded. I shrug. "It's not that big of a deal. Plus, they're probably watching their other Test Tube Baby, since they're not allowed to bring them in."

I space out watching an older woman in the reception kiosk put on her morning makeup at her desk. Orson and I wonder if we'll both have to be on fertility meds at the same time and if we'll lose our minds.

"I think we should write letters to each other, before we start the meds," I say. "Like, 'Dear Orson, Please remember how sweet and loving I am to you when not on fertility drugs. Please recall how mostly in control of my emotions I am. Please do not break up with me.' Things like that. Letters to ourselves might be helpful, too: 'Dear Self. None of this is real. You are crazy. Go sit by yourself, or sob in the shower. Leave Orson alone.'"

A student resident who is not lesbionic Jan brings us to Dr. Waller, who stands up behind his desk and offers his hand to Orson. They shake. It's love at first sight. There's something in Dr. Waller's Jewish swagger that Orson takes to immediately, and as for Dr. Waller, well, how often does he get a patient like Orson? A young, dapper man-woman bequeathing a precious egg to their beloved?

"Okay," Dr. Waller says, with a glint in his wire-rimmed eyes. "Let's talk about this. We're using *your* eggs." Dr. Waller points his pen at Orson. "Am I right?"

Orson nods. I feel that Orson is probably biting back a "yes, sir."

"Well, that should not be a problem, then." Dr. Waller smiles at Orson. "What we'll see on your ultrasound today isn't the eggs, because the eggs are too small, right? What we can see is the *fluid* the eggs are living inside. Each month one egg outgrows the rest, and that's the egg that gets ovulated. That one egg suppresses the rest of them, and the others die off."

Wait. Wait a second! This is big information! The whole narrative around conception is always about that *one* sperm—the mighty, hardy, fastest, luckiest sperm that outraces all the other sperms and grabs on to the long blond weave of the Rapunzel egg sitting passively in her castle and—BAM—bores into her mightily and knocks her up! This half-assed factoid has laid the foundation of a millennia of misogyny, casting men as active go-getters and women as passive and fragile.

How is it that I am forty-one years old and I am just now learning that there is a race to the death happening inside my body every month? That some intense Alpha Egg is growing silently inside of me, indistinguishable from all the others until the day she just surges ahead, stealing the life-force from her sisters, buffing up to make the trip down the fallopian highway?

I wonder what sort of psychic difference it would make on our culture *and* on individual females if that metaphor-rich bit of information was common knowledge. Think of the billions of competitive scenarios, the close calls, the moments when the underdog suddenly bursts forth with a special talent and slays the competition. All can be likened to the Egg, biding its time until it harnesses its strength and wipes out the playing field. I can't wait to have a kid so I can teach them all about this stuff.

"Your brain sends out FSH, follicle-stimulating hormone, and this causes all the eggs to start to grow," Dr. Waller continues. "But something stops that procedure once that one egg begins to dominate. The meds we give you will override that, so *many* eggs will grow toward ovulation." Orson will inject these meds every day for two weeks. "You'll take a class to learn how," says Dr. Waller, and Orson looks at me quickly with a pleading face.

"I'll give you the injections," I say. We'll both be taking that class.

During the weeks that Orson is getting shot up with their eggs-ellent medications, they'll also be coming in four or five times for ultrasounds and blood draws. I'm scribbling everything into my notebook as fast as the doctor says it, but my pen stops when he spits the term *gonadotropin.* These fertility drugs are called gonado-tropins, because guess what? They stimulate the *gonads,* which in my body and maybe yours are known also as *ovaries.* Yeah, that's right—women have got gonads, too! All these years of feeling emasculated by the spin that science has put on my bod, thinking that only men had nads, thereby having "the nads" to do all sorts of brave and foolish things. Harrumph.

Dr. Waller continues detailing how modern medicine will over-ride Orson's natural system. On day fourteen of Orson's synthe-sized cycle, they will get a dose of LH—luteinizing hormone, the hormone that will make all the eggs head for the uterus. Thirty-six hours later, the doctor will go in and snag them via a vaginal probe.

I hate the thought of Orson being in pain, which is why I am relieved to hear Dr. Waller say that they'll be put in a "twilight" state for the egg retrieval. They'll get these beautiful, wonderful, luxurious drugs that will slip them into a lovely drugged-out state and make it seem like nothing at all happened.

Dr. Waller moves on to discuss the ups and downs of frozen sperm. When I bring up the possibility of using Quentin's sperm, he shoots it down. He says what a lot of people say: that it's a really big deal, the life we are bringing into existence, and even though people seem really cool with it at the start, things can change, people have feelings, things get very complicated, there are *grand-parents* involved for god's sake, and if we are just trying to start a family together, we're better off using an anonymous donor from a sperm bank.

I get what he's saying, and maybe I'm naïve, but I really in my heart believe that Quentin would never pose a problem with our kid. I also know that I'd be into Quentin having a relationship with the kid if he ever wants that. As far as an extended family, I don't know. My family is pretty small and so is Orson's. I think the more love and support a kid gets in their lives, the better. But it doesn't matter, because the amount of money and logistical nightmares it would take to use Quentin's sperm seems to mean that a bank would be the best route for us, anyway. I feel a real disappointment ring through my body at the thought of losing Quentin. I love him, I love his *genes,* I love his generosity, I love what his presence does to this story of procreation. I guess I am really drawn to the less traditional, queer, and community-centric mode of making a family, and less interested in the type of fortress a normal nuclear family tends to be. Don't we all know by now how problematic nuclear families are, and how everything is made better by the presence of queerness? How were we going to replace the truly irreplaceable Quentin with some boring straight dude? I snap myself out of the blah mood such thoughts put me in. After all, the real point here is to have a baby. And Dr. Waller is just trying to show us the path toward that dream.

It's time for the doctor to play *Asteroids* with Orson's junk. We're escorted into the tiny room where I once lay with my own feet in stirrups, and are left alone for Orson to strip below the waist and climb onto the exam table. They place a paper blanket over their hips and set their feet in the stirrups. They look at me and smile.

"I know this makes a beautiful picture," they say, "but you can't take it."

I smile back. "Are you sure you're okay?" I ask them. They nod. Then they see the wand. "Oh jeez, is *that* what's going in me?"

Looking at the wand, I am suddenly reminded of a David Shrigley show we just saw. The artist is obsessed with eerily long fingers and both draws them and sculpts them.

"Doesn't that look like one of David Shrigley's fingers?" I ask.

"I was wondering why it looked sort of familiar!"

I get up close to the machine and notice a bag of giant condoms. "Look," I say.

"We aren't normal," Orson says, shaking their head. "We do things in special ways."

Dr. Waller knocks and enters. "Okay, you got your feety in the feety holders," he quips. I cringe on Orson's behalf as he inserts a condom-covered Shrigley finger into their junk and begins to wiggle the wand around to get the best view of their insides.

"Now, that is a *really* good-looking ovary," he says cheerfully. Orson beams with pride. "Go on, take a look," the doctor offers.

I lean over Orson and peer at the tiny, wet-looking circles glistening in black and white on the screen. It's Orson's eggs! One of those could be our kid! I almost tear up thinking it, and then remember that one of those innocent-looking microscopic donuts is going to rise up and murder the others.

"Okay, we're done," says the doctor. We're all satisfied with the pronouncement of Orson's ovaries as "good-looking." The doctor leaves and Orson hops off the table.

"That was kind of fun!" they exclaim before I can even ask them how they're doing.

"You like an adventure." I laugh. "And you like science. It's like your own scientific experiment on yourself."

Back in Dr. Waller's office, he continues with the endless details of how all of this will go down. "So, you have about eighteen eggs in there," he tells Orson. "With ovary stimulation, we should get about sixteen eggs," he says. "And I could be underestimating you." Orson beams again. Their ovaries *rule*.

"Let's just say we're gonna get sixteen eggs. Odds are, thirteen of them will be mature. Eight will fertilize. We'll grow those eight embryos for five days."

"Like, in a test tube?" Orson asks.

"Yes." He nods. "Maybe four will make it. We'll transfer the best-looking one, and we'll freeze the other three. If it doesn't work, we'll transfer another."

"So, if the best one doesn't work, you use one of the lousy ones?" Orson says, half joking.

"You might have two equal ones," he says. "With your eggs, we have an incredibly high success rate. My *conservative* guess would be a sixty to eighty percent likelihood of success."

Those odds are *so* much better than the odds of my scraggly eggs! And the whole tone of this meeting is so much better—more optimistic, with talk of good-looking eggs and high success rates, not the funeral drum that played at my own appointment. I feel excited! I feel like it's *safe* to get excited. Nothing makes it easier to imagine spending your entire savings than the phrase "incredibly high success rate."

13.

SUPERMODELS, ATHLETES, AND PREGNANT WOMEN

There is so much information to gather and assimilate at Dr. Waller's office. Orson is going to have to get some lab work done, testing for infectious diseases, checking their hormone levels, plus a special peep at their genetics to see if, as an Ashkenazi Jew, they are a carrier of Tay-Sachs disease.

As for me, I'm to have a saline sonogram to make sure my womb is spick-and-span, and then it's onward to Babymakingsville! Orson and I will be put on hormones to synch our cycles. We'll get calendars! Each tiny square of time will list what meds we're to take that day, which injections and patches and pills, one for me, one for Orson.

I'll be given estrogen to thicken my uterine lining, then proges-terone to hold on to the baby. Orson will be given chemicals to make their ovaries produce all the eggs.

Dr. Waller tells us to register for the monthly IVF orientations. I imagine a mixer, with couples spun out on a heady mixture of financial dread, optimistic desperation, and general infertility ennui drifting about, knocking back folic acid with glasses of sparkling water, preemptively avoiding the soft cheese plate.

"Now, your ovaries are going to get really big," Dr. Waller warns Orson. "You'll feel bloated. And there are small risks to everything, just like walking down the street." What he is telling us is fewer than 1 percent of the people getting Orson's injections get ovarian hyperstimulation syndrome.

"Your ovaries start going haywire like a chicken," he tells us. "They produce *lots* of eggs, and the eggs send blood to other parts of the body . . ." He shakes his head at the mess of it. "There's the potential to be hospitalized." I think about how orderly and organized, how controlled and thoughtful Orson is. It would be totally unlike them, energetically, to have such spazzy, unruly ovaries.

"Is there an emotional side effect to the ovarian stimulation?" they ask the doctor. Yeah, who cares about berserk ovaries, we want to know if we'll have any *real* problems, like feeling crazy and crying all the time.

"No," he says. "You're going to feel bloated and maybe those pants won't fit you that well."

Orson goes on to share another concern, that if the sperm donor has successfully fertilized other eggs, then our kid might have siblings walking around. What if they accidentally date each other or something?

"Thank god there's a billion people in the world," Dr. Waller says, and shrugs. I look at Orson like, *Do you fucking love this guy or what?*

Finally, we are freed from the doctor's office. As we wait for the elevator, I point out the little chair by the window, the little table holding a box of Kleenex. "It's the crying chair," I whisper. "That's where I called you from when I learned my eggs were busted."

We wait until we are out of the sort of hushed and somber women's health building before exploding with excitement on the street.

"Isn't Dr. Waller great?" I demand.

"I love him! I really love him!"

"I know, he's so excellent! He said you have *good-looking ovaries*. That is the best compliment ever."

"I think he loves us," Orson says, nodding with insight. "I think he really loves us."

"I bet he does!" I cry. "We're his quirky lesbian patients!"

As if on cue, Orson's phone rings. They look at the screen; the number looks vaguely familiar. "I think it might be the clinic," I say. "Answer it."

Orson picks up and the loud, slightly East Coast timbre of Dr. Waller's voice is streaming muffled through the phone. They talk for a moment and Orson hangs up. They are beaming from this extra contact with the doctor, who they are perhaps now in love with.

"What'd he say?"

"He said he tried to get our psychiatric evaluation waived. He doesn't think we should have to do it."

"Right, because we shouldn't!" I get steamed about it right away. "It's totally homophobic. This is how lesbians utilize a fertility clinic. If a male partner doesn't have to get counseled before giving his wife some sperm, you shouldn't have to get counseled around giving me your egg!"

Alas, it's procedure for a "woman" "donating" her egg to undergo a counseling session—Dr. Waller's efforts fail. I pledge to protest it every step of the way, complain my butt off to whomever I can, and to make the session an entertaining pain-in-the-ass for the unfortunate counselor. So much to look forward to!

Orson is on cloud nine for the rest of the day. Not even the specter of a homophobic counseling session can ruin the joy of learning that their ovaries rule and that our doctor is rad.

I CALL MY SISTER, MADELINE, TO TELL HER HOW IT WENT. "SIXTY TO EIGHTY PERCENT success rate!" I cry. "That is so much better than my elderly eggs!"

"Know what my doctor told me when I was going in for all my high-risk-pregnancy tests?" she asks. "The only people considered 'old' at thirty-eight are supermodels, athletes, and pregnant women. You're not elderly."

"I know I'm not," I agree. The weird thing is, I am in better health and spirits than I ever have been in my whole entire life. Finally, at forty-one, I am in a stable relationship. I'm financially stable. Thanks to my meds, I'm emotionally stable. I'm almost ten years sober. It's crazy that now, during this phase of my life, when I am most suited to have kids, my body is over it. I decide that if we have a daughter, we're going to get her eggs frozen when she's eighteen, so she can run around and have international lovers and become a big career woman or run herself into the ground making performance art or live life in whatever baby-free way she'd like to spend her twenties. Then she can have herself a baby if and whenever she wants, because the uterus, amazingly, does not really age. Your uterus is just as good for childbirth in your fifties as it is in your twenties. Isn't that unbelievable? Only the eggs go bad. Things are going to be different for our little girl!

Meeting with Dr. Waller was a big marker on our baby pathway. The next one? My fibroid surgery, which was set to take place the following week. A few things will be happening during my surgery recovery. Our new couch will be delivered. The cable guy will install cable. And we will be visited by Fleabusters, a company which claims to kill fleas dead by applying some solution that dehydrates the little fuckers to death all over your home. Fleabusters say they'll come back and kill them again if they don't die the first time, though they assure you they *will*, they *will* die the first time. Though it is perhaps slightly insane that all of these things will be happening while I am recovering from surgery, I am thrilled that they are happening. I am thrilled to be living with Orson, and the wild circumstances surrounding it don't even bother me.

For my surgery, I wear a cute, long-sleeved denim dress I got on sale for $19.99. The dress is perfect because it won't bother my belly and also because it will add much balancing cute energy to my post-surgery aura, which I expect to be pasty and spooky. At the hospital, they rip me away from Orson far too soon. Everything is kind of cloudy in my memory—*probably because I was drugged and sedated to the brink of death!* The operating room was large and gray, with crazy operating contraptions like miniature cranes, and there was some smooth jazz playing softly in the background. (Isn't that funny? Doctors and nurses like to listen to music while they work, just like cabdrivers and baristas.) I was already getting woozy when Dr. Becky walked up and said hi. *Of course* Dr. Becky would be wearing her head covering at a jaunty angle, like a beret. I'm so happy to see her, it's like she's my best friend, and she actually *holds my hand* while I wait to go under. That's my last memory— Dr. Becky holding my hand, smiling down at me, maybe even tenderly rubbing my palm.

I wake up in my room after the surgery, and Orson is there. "Dr. Becky held my hand," I croak. And I regale them with the other new info: not only was my bod "riddled" with fibroids, as Dr. Waller so charmingly put it, but the Queen Fibroid, according to Dr. Becky, was "as big as a baby's head. Bigger."

"I don't think many women feel that different after these surgeries," she had told me. "But I think you might." And I do. Once my swelling goes down and my body returns to normal, I find that I actually do feel much lighter, and the weird heavy feeling I had was gone.

But before my body returns to normal, I have been instructed to lie around in bed, popping pills. As an addict, I am excited for the possibilities of this freelapse, but mostly the pills just keep the pain at bay so I can function in my life. But the more drugs I put in my system, the more a weird tinge begins to spread. One night, after Orson spends about twenty minutes rubbing my shoulders, I try to get them to get it on with me. Pills always make me amorous (when not putting me into a blackout). Let's imagine how appealing I am—surgery breath, scabby belly, pasty skin, matted hair, pill-sweat on my pajamas. Brave Orson makes out with me a little, but puts the brakes on when I tried to go to third base.

"Baby, you just had surgery," they say gently.

I burst into tears. "You don't love me!" I wail. I'm pretty sure I accuse them of doing nothing to help me, though they had only just given me a massage and had been bringing me Kozy Shack Chocolate Pudding after Kozy Shack Chocolate Pudding for forty-eight hours. I sob so hard, you would think I had just witnessed a major humanitarian tragedy. I soak a hankie with viscous snot, becoming even more grotesque. I want a cigarette *so bad*.

Oh yeah—when I take drugs, *I cry*! Toward the end of my using, that was all that ever happened. And just like everyone in 12-step says, all that time you're sober, not drinking or using, your addiction is still there inside you. It progresses, even though you're not feeding it anymore. It doesn't go away. I remember a guy at a meeting in Brooklyn, saying in a perfect New York accent, "My addiction is downstairs in the basement, doing push-ups." Totally! I go into the bathroom and weep loudly, hoping the sound of my pain is tearing Orson's heart apart.

The next day I am horrified. It is like I had gone on a very deep bender. I hate that Orson—who has never seen me drunk—has seen me in such a condition. It is like the space-time continuum tore and horrid 2002 Michelle fell into 2012 Michelle's perfect life. I decide not to take the pills anymore. Fuck it. People have all sorts of procedures and don't take painkillers; alcoholics in 12-step talk about it all the time. It isn't worth it to them, getting so close to those dangerous old feelings.

I try that for a day and finally feel what it *really* is like to have a robot chew your fibroids up. It is as if a Norwegian black metal drummer has mistaken me for his drum set. Like I've gone to Great America and spent the day lying down on various coaster tracks. I feel tremendously bad. I start taking the pills again, warning both Orson and myself to ignore any feelings I might claim to be having. None of them are real. And if they are, they can wait till I am off the Vicodin to process them.

In bed on the pills, flipping through fashion magazines, I get a call and it's my sister. She's had her baby! A little boy named Aiden, a Leo. Maddy sounds happy and lonely, hormonal and sweet. We talk on the phone for a bit, each in our respective recovery beds, each on our meds, all for the sake of having babies. The text photos start pouring in, and the baby is beautiful, he looks just like her daughter, Olivia, and my sister and my brother-in-law, Walden. Olivia is psyched about her baby brother and soon takes to yelling in his face, "AIDEN! Are you lookin' at your big sister?" I do my Weird Aunt duties and pull up his chart on the internet. All Leo and Aries. He's going to be a lady-killer! Or a man-killer! Or whatever! (I actually hate more than *anything* when people are like, "Ooooh, he/she loves the ladies/boys, he/she is such a flirt, is that your new girlfriend/boyfriend" about their INFANTS. But his astrological chart *does* predict he'll be a bit of a Casanova.)

Orson joins me in bed to ooh and aah at the pictures of tiny Aiden, and we resume our conversation about sperm. In the abstract, all there is to talk about is ethnicity, which is a little weird, but we go for it. My big idea is to highlight all of Orson's most elfin characteristics with some Icelandic sperm. I know we're supposed to be finding sperm that matches my own ethnic heritage, right, but really, I'm not too jazzed about my people. I'm from New England, home of Irish pride, which looks like an angry, drunk, red-faced, red-haired racist dude in a "Fightin' Irish" baseball hat. And Polish? What does Polish even look like? I imagine if we could somehow get sperm from, say, Björk, that's what I would like.

Orson is against the Icelandic sperm idea. They think searching out some general European mutt sperm is our best bet. Maybe it's the pills, but I feel moody and irritated about having to pick out sperm at all. If we just naturally created a baby between us and it was Polish because I am Polish, I'd be like, whatever, that's how it goes. I wouldn't think so much about it. Going out of your way to pick European sperm, or non-European sperm, it all feels creepy. I wish there was a way to play sperm roulette.

That night, on the computer, I google "best sperm bank." The most compelling and well-reviewed place is the lesbian-owned joint right here in San Francisco. I download a PDF that breaks their donors down into the most rudimentary stats. Even so, I find myself totally sucked into the lines of type. A Peruvian soccer player who likes music and photography? Sounds cool! A European mutt with my entire ethnic makeup plus some Nicaraguan blood? Awesome! For the first time since turning away from my True Love Donor, Quentin, I feel a little excitement about sperm choices. I shut my computer before I get carried away, eager to share my findings with Orson.

14.

THERE ARE LESBIANS

I t's time for our IVF orientation. I imagined being very bored. I did not imagine being greeted by a wide table laden with snacks. Of course there are snacks: when you spend a bunch of money somewhere, they are pretty much obligated to feed you. I pile my plate high, with that desperate feeling I get around free things surging through me.

A smiling woman approaches as I build a massive cheese-and-fruit pyramid on my plate and hands me a bound handbook titled *IVF Orientation*. That little part of me that always feels like it never belongs anywhere thinks that maybe they'll think I'm just an IVF orientation crasher, here to scam some food. Do I look like a person who can afford this? This isn't a dull meeting in a cramped conference room. It's a nominally catered event held in a theater. Trying to stop grapes from rolling off my plate, I follow Orson into the venue.

Immediately, I see a lez couple, and they see me, and we exchange a really cute, *Hey, we're lesbians having test tube babies* smile of camaraderie. Orson and I hike up to the back and take our seats. I can't wait to show them the lesbians.

"Orson, there are lesbians!" I hiss. "Did you see them?"

"Um, those ones right there?" they hiss in an even quieter hissy voice, pointing to the seats directly in front of us. We are facing the back of a short, butch haircut seated beside the back of a longer, femme hairdo pinned up in the back with a claw.

WOW, I mouth silently. I point down to the dykes in the front whom I smiled at. I then realize one of them attends the same 12-step program I do. Double awesome. The orientation is shaping up nicely, though ultimately the queer presence is pretty small.

The orientation has the form of a lecture, and tonight's will be delivered by a Dr. Murakami and none other than Dr. Waller. Orson and I look at each other and smile proudly. There are probably about twelve doctors working in the clinic, so it feels special that ours is delivering the information tonight.

Dr. Murakami is up first. He is in hard-core teacher mode, immediately disappointed with us for not participating. I remember this is a teaching hospital, and he probably stands there a few times a week addressing eager students antsy to outsmart one another and impress their teacher. Not this crowd. This crowd is a bunch of middle-aged heterosexuals tired from eight hours at their J.O.B., exhausted by their pregnancy fails, scared and nervous, hopeful and overwhelmed by what they are stepping into. No one is optimistically raising their hands to answer Dr. Murakami's questions.

The doctor catches on to this, and switches tactics, brings up some issues we might be collectively having. "There can be feelings of depression and anxiety." He clicks a clicker, and a picture of the infernal in-house psychologist we have to have our dumb session with pops onto the screen. The psychologist does look a little eccentric. Maybe it won't be too bad, but I still resent it.

"There is a high risk of loss of pregnancy in the population we serve." Dr. Murakami explores the myriad of reasons we all feel so bummed out, then moves quickly to the science, the nuts and bolts of what will happen to our bodies.

Orson and I are already pretty well versed in this thanks to our meeting with Dr. Waller, but it is amusing to hear Dr. Murakami explain it all. "Do any of you surf?" he excitedly queries the crowd. "No? Okay. Think of all the eggs in the ovaries as surfers. When one surfer catches the wave, the other surfers are eliminated. With IVF, all the surfers catch the wave!" Prior to the surfer metaphor, I had been trying to refrain from psychotic note-taking, but I *had* to get this down. I let go and furiously scribble the surfing metaphor onto my napkin.

There is a lot of talk about how the doctors will "rescue" the eggs via the medicines and procedures. The eggs aren't really being rescued, because they are not *meant* to survive, so the language makes the doctors sound sort of benevolent and heroic, rather than subverters of the natural rhythms of the female body.

A picture of an egg gets flashed onto the screen. It looks like a flower, or a sunburst. The egg is in the center of a web of cells Dr. Murakami likens to worker bees, situating the egg as queen. The cells feed the egg, and they also catch and trap any sperm, keeping it close to the egg.

"Out of ten eggs, one will fertilize." He shares the grim statistic, then introduces a new slide of a fertilized egg. It looks like a meringue.

The doctors fertilize the eggs and then watch them for six days, making sure they develop nicely. Whichever one looks best by day five gets implanted. By day six, the embryo splits into what looks like two distinct cells.

"It's up to the embryo to implant," Dr. Murakami says. Some embryos just keep drifting along, right back up the fallopian tubes and, whammo, you got yourself an ectopic pregnancy. Even a natural fertilization process can lead to such a scenario, but the risk is higher with IVF.

Dr. Murakami pulls up a slide of percentages. The age of the egg will determine the likelihood of a successful IVF. Orson is in "Below 34" range, the top percentage, lumped in with freaking sixteen-year-olds! I feel so grateful and also burning with urgency. They'll turn thirty-three next month. This is our year.

The PowerPoint presentation flips to a new slide, illustrated with a snowman. "We have a big problem with 'orphan embryos,'" Dr. Murakami says. "They are embryos that have been abandoned by the parents. Once they're stored, they can outlive you. It is why we are now so anal about making you consent to what you will do with the embryos."

Dr. Murakami clicks off his neon green laser pointer and drops it into the pocket of his lab coat. It's time for Dr. Waller to take the stage, to talk about sperm. When Dr. Waller talks about the sperm—getting the sperm to the eggs and all that, letting them swim to it, that one hardy sperm who breaks through and fertilizes—he uses army metaphors. People always use army metaphors for sperm and it bums me out. I don't want something traumatic and terrible like colonialism to be associated with the birth of our darling offspring who may grow up and *cure war!* But also, being out of my element makes me defensive and I take refuge in radicalism. Orson, who mostly had a boy's childhood, playing army with their siblings, thinks it's sort of cute. They are clearly thinking of toys and playtime and perhaps hard work and ambition, while I am thinking of genocide.

Dr. Waller cues up a three-minute video of a blastomere biopsy. We are treated to a quick image of a needle sliding into and sucking away a piece of a blastocyst, which is basically an egg that's been fertilized for like four days. I guess they'll do a biopsy before implantation if they think the embryo could be at risk for things like Huntington's disease, sickle cell, hemophilia, and situations concerning sex hormones. Or if the IVF hasn't been working.

Orson and I gasp watching the video—it's just so weird and cool. "We're embryo nerds!" I whisper. "This is like being in med school! I'm so into it!"

"Me too!" Orson smiles.

"Don't you want to go home and watch episodes of *NOVA* and eat Oreos?" I beg.

"Totally."

The final slide in the PowerPoint presentation is titled "A Healthy Singleton"—the ideal end result for all of us, except the baby is freaking ugly.

"That's an ugly baby," Orson whispers.

"Ugs," I confirm.

Dr. Waller talks about the magical uterus. "The uterus is an amazing organ that stays the same age," he says. "Twenty or fifty, it's the same." He does bring up fibroids and polyps and how those can get in the way. "It's not uncommon, though it is the minority," he says. "Twenty to twenty-five percent." Hmph. I always knew I was special.

Dr. Waller opens the floor for questions, and a lady raises her hand to ask if she can please be implanted with two embryos, because she would like to have two kids and it would be easier to do it all at once. Easier—and cheaper! I see through this crazy hustler's scheme.

Dr. Waller shakes his head emphatically. The clinic will most certainly *not* be giving anyone twins, at least not on purpose. "Humans in general were not meant to carry twins," he says. "Plus, you try for twins and you get triplets. Can't do it."

The orientation is over. We want to say hello to Dr. Waller—am I crazy, or has he spotted us out of the corner of his eye and is now politely trying to wrap it up with some boring dude so he can spend a minute with us, his favorite patients? We'll never know. After lingering awkwardly for a moment, we join the flow of people leaving the lecture hall and go home. I feel a little dazed from the onslaught of information, detached from being outside my comfort zone, and a little embarrassed by how deep in it we really are, *artificial reproductive technology*, something I swore I'd never do. But sloshing around this mixture of emotion is another one, pearly and sweet. I feel hopeful.

15.

I'M AN AQUARIUS

The biggest allure of using sperm bank sperm, especially for Orson, is the idea that no one else is involved in our family. It's just us—Mom, Baba, and Baby. It provides an illusion of control. In reality, four people will have come together in this family.

A study from 2005 run in Oxford Academic's publication *Human Reproduction* reports that 80 percent of surveyed donor kids aged twelve to seventeen want to meet their biological father. I totally get this. If I grew up without knowing who my dad was, I would be completely, utterly obsessed. I've become fanatical about family mysteries that aren't even that interesting. An unknown father? I'd be fantasizing that he was rich, famous, an artist, a genius, the key to everything about myself that ever mystified me. He'd be the balm for every wound inflicted by my parents—whenever they didn't understand me properly, or seemed to be working against me, I'd be like, "I bet my *dad* would get me/let me stay out all night/know how stupid this rule is." I know myself enough to know this one hundred percent. And I know I'm not that unique in the world.

What were the chances that our sperm bank donor, when he enters our life eighteen years from now, will be even a *fraction* as adorable, sweet, generous, creative, intelligent, politically radical, stylish, and gay as Quentin? I'd say the chances were less than zero. I became filled with urgent energy. We just had to use Quentin's sperm, no matter the cost. It was just too important.

I send Orson an intense sperm donor email, full of anecdotes and statistics that suggest we're doing our future kid a disservice by going through a sperm bank.

"I'm really open to following your lead with this," they say after reading. "I think you're being very wise about it." Ultimately, it's about community. The community we are creating for our child to live inside. "I trust Quentin one hundred," Orson says, "but I'd want to have a conversation."

Truthfully, I didn't have much of a conversation with Quentin when we started "working together," i.e., when he began coming over my house and jerking off into a warm bowl in my kitchen. I go more on vibes, trust, and optimism, and while this sounds admittedly shaky, it has served me well. Orson, though—they want structure, information, order. Which totally makes sense, especially for such a big deal as a baby. They're also a worrier, sniffing out potential bad scenes that never really occur to me.

"What about Quentin's parents?" they ask. "What if they want to spend time with their grandkid?"

I think most people who find out they have grandkids would be pretty obsessed with meeting them and spending time with them. Quentin's family background feels familiar to Orson—Jewish and middle class, kind, family-oriented. Orson thinks they are for sure going to want to claim our baby as their grandkid. From what I know of them, gleaned mostly through photos Quentin has shared of the over-the-top holiday decorating his mother indulges in, I agree. My mother is an over-the-top holiday decorator as well, and I think that people who enjoy putting snowmen figurines all over the house each winter are also the kind of people who want to spoil a grandkid.

But truthfully, this doesn't concern me very much. If there are another few people in the world who want to love our kid and look out for them, I think that's great.

"We won't owe them anything, not any more than we owe our own parents," I say. "But chances are they'd be great."

Orson nods. "I know these people," they confirm. "I'm sure they are wonderful."

As scary as it is to know we don't have complete control over the creation of our little family, I think it's a blessing. Really, no one has control over their families, or over anything. The situations that make that clear to us, though often hard, are blessings in the long run.

"Thank you for being so open and so sweet-hearted about this," I tell Orson. "Should I make a dinner date with Quentin?"

"Just give me a couple days to think about it," they say, slowing me down. "You just want to *go*, don't you?"

"I do!" I say.

"We have some time," Orson says. I like to rush into everything wildly, and Orson likes to be a slowpoke. I think they help me rein it in, and I help light a fire under their butt. It's a good compromise for both of us.

I toggle between popcorn and Oreos, eating my feelings. Soon we will pack Rodney into a rental car and drive down to Southern California to spend Christmas with my sister and her family. We agree to put off the Quentin decision until we return.

16.

WE'RE BETTER THAN THIS

Christmas is spent in Los Angeles, celebrating with Maddy and Walden, Olivia and baby Aiden. My mom comes out from Florida. Walden's mother, a glamorous retired TV exec, spoils us rotten with a decadent meal at a restaurant that faces the Pacific Ocean. Through the window, the waves come in, and come in again, hitting the shore, hitting the shore, hitting the shore. I don't know what their endgame is, these waves, but I'll take from them their focus, their steady repetition, their inability to give up. We're both controlled by the moon, after all. At dinner, there is no talk of babies not born, not when we've got the newbie Aiden to coo at. But back at Maddy's house, when everyone is asleep but us sisters, chatting late into the night, she asks me how it's going, and I tell her of our plan to once again ask Quentin for his sperm. I don't know what he'll say; maybe he's truly exhausted from nearly a year of epic monthly inseminations. And it's hard to say if this next era of trying, with the help of the Fertility Industrial Complex, will be easier or more complicated for him.

Back in San Francisco, Orson and I take Quentin to brunch at a fancy place out in Dogpatch, a slowly gentrifying, once-industrial part of San Francisco, and ask him if he's up for returning to Donorsville. All my worries were for naught.

"Of course!" he says, smiling.

For Orson's benefit, Quentin reiterates his deep lack of interest in having anything to do with raising our kid *and* his openness to the kid knowing that they're spawned from his glittering seed. Orson shares their grandparent concerns, but Quentin is not telling his parents about this. Not now, maybe someday. We make it clear that we're not *asking* him not to tell them. We can't really ask such things of Quentin. But it sounds like he's not currently available for the feelings avalanche such news would surely bring down either.

We drop Quentin back at the house where he's staying. Quentin has moved to Santa Cruz for grad school, but is keeping a large drag closet in San Francisco for his weekend performances. The drag closet has a mattress, so he crashes there and then returns to the coast, where he buzzes around town on a cute green Vespa. Quentin is so adorable it makes me want to *die*. Or have his baby.

IT'S NEW YEAR'S EVE. NEXT WEEK I'LL HAVE A FINAL SONOGRAM TO GET THE ALL-clear on my womb, and then it's just about getting Quentin set up at the clinic. I'm super ready to celebrate our awesome *life!* We decide to go karaoke in a private room to ring in 2013, joined by Vito, who is in town with his girlfriend, Liza. Mel joins us, as does Vito's cousin Floridana, whom Mel has been making out with.

We get to the karaoke room first, which is *great,* because that means I can try out a couple of iffy numbers before a real audience arrives. Orson immediately orders a pitcher of beer and a giant bottle of sake, seemingly ignorant of what a ridiculous amount of booze this is. Soon, our friends arrive, right in the middle of me attempting the falsetto heights of Def Leppard's "Bringing on the

Heartache." Orson forces a beer on Mel. Floridana shows up and pours some sake. Vito starts programming a barrage of songs into the queue, and we're off!

We had the room reserved for two hours. Two hours is *not* enough time in a karaoke room. We beg for another hour, and it's granted. Meanwhile, Orson is getting drunk. Mel is getting drunk. Floridana is getting drunk. I'm sober as ever, but enjoying the fun-house vibe my friends' inebriation is giving off. Sometimes it's enjoyable to be around drunk people. When that hour ends, we add yet another.

While two hours is not long enough in a karaoke room, four hours is too much. Orson is so drunk they're forgetting what songs they've put into the queue. They flub the lyrics to Pulp songs they could sing in their sleep. Mel's initial greeting was too warm for the hot-and-cold Floridana, so the two of *them* sit across the room from each other, emitting strange vibes. Floridana is drunk and wild, singing brassy show tunes. Mel is drunk and morose, climbing on the benches to sing Echo and the Bunnymen at the wall, or lying down on the floor like they have given up on life. Vito, who takes karaoke *way* too seriously, is becoming aggro. It's a lesson in leaving the party when you're having fun. By the time we leave the party, the fun has sort of leaked away, and it's not even midnight.

Vito has decided to lead us all to a church on a hill to see the fireworks at midnight. As we walk along, I realize how *wasted* Orson is. They want to go to a party at Tali and Bernadine's house, but I keep explaining it's *not* a party, it's just Tali and Bernadine and one other couple filling out these introspective, 12-steppy workbooks. There is no way I can bring wasted Orson into their quiet observation of 2013.

Orson gets offended at this, the way people who are very drunk can get offended when someone points out that they are in fact very drunk. Orson insists they're not drunk.

"Well, you're too drunk to go over to Tali's," I say. Tali is sober and sensitive to drunks.

"Listen," Orson tries to reason with me. "Pretend you just met me. Okay?"

"Okay," I say, knowing this is only something a drunk person would propose to prove they're not drunk.

"Hi," they say.

"Hello," I say back.

"See?" they say.

The obsession with crashing Tali's sober domesticity is forgotten as a cab cruises by, and Orson jumps into it without saying goodbye to anyone. I'm actually sick of walking and want to go home, so I'm grateful for the cab and leap in next to Orson, shouting a goodbye to everyone else

It is mostly fun being with drunk Orson, because they're so silly. But then there are moments when they don't understand what I'm saying and go, "What did you say?" in a sort of defensive way that reminds me that they're drunk and that drunk people are volatile. At home we go up to the roof to watch the fireworks.

"You have to be very, very careful," I tell them as we begin our ascent up four flights of stairs to our roof.

"I'm fine," they say, smashing into an aluminum ladder hanging on a hook outside a neighbor's door.

On the roof, the fireworks are awesome explosions in the foggy darkness. We hug and watch them twinkle and fade, then get a little bored and go downstairs.

"I'll make us a frozen pizza," I tell them. "And why don't you take some ibuprofen?"

"I don't want to take any ibuprofen," they snap.

I've seen Orson suffer a hangover from a couple of beers; I know they are going to be clobbered tomorrow. "Just take a couple and have some water," I urge them. "You'll be really glad you did in the morning."

"I said I don't *want* to, and I don't like being *forced* to take medicine."

"Really?" I ask, truly baffled. "You don't want to just not have a hangover tomorrow?"

Orson grows more incensed and claims that it's *dangerous* for them to take ibuprofen while drinking. They say it in a deeply offended tone, like I am trying to kill them. Now we're arguing.

"Orson, you don't want to do this," I tell them. "Let's just forget it, okay?"

I go into the kitchen and make a slab of frozen pizza. I know they are going to feel like *such* a fool in the morning, but my feelings are stinging and so are my eyes. I hate being talked to like that. I get myself together and bring the pizza into the bed, where we eat it side by side in silence.

"Really?" I ask. "We're just going to sit here and not talk to each other?"

Apparently, we are. What about the superstition about how you spend New Year's Eve is how you're doomed to spend the entire year? I'm sad and hurt and angry and can't believe we are having a fight about taking ibuprofen. We're better than this.

"You know, it's really easy to blame the drunk person, because they can't defend themselves," Orson mutters.

I decide the moment is bad enough to justify me dredging my pack of Secret Cigarettes out of the junk drawer to smoke in the yard. I hop out of bed. Orson responds with alarm.

"Where are you going?"

"To the yard."

They know what that means. It breaks their heart.

"No, no, no, you can't!" they cry. "Please, please get in bed with me!"

Normal Orson has fought their way through drunk, belligerent Orson. I get back in the bed, and Orson wraps themself around me, crying. They ask if I'm going to leave them. I laugh.

"No," I tell them. "I'm never going to leave you."

In the morning things feel delicate. We kiss and hug and eat croissants and Orson calls me into the living room for a surprise. They have a big wrapped present for me.

"What is this?" I ask, delighted. "Christmas is over!"

"Just open it."

I unwrap what is the greatest jewelry box. It's a maroon leather case with drawers that slide out and reveal more secret drawers.

"Keep going, look at all the compartments," they urge.

I pull out the last drawer, which holds a tray divided for rings and earrings. For a moment I don't understand the diamond ring that is sitting there on a tawny velveteen pillow. And then I do, and my body flushes hot and cold, a totally physical sensation, numb and rushing at once. And Orson is talking, they're telling me that they love me so much and they want to take care of me forever and will I marry them, and I am crying and touching the diamond—which I never, ever thought I'd give a fuck about, a diamond, who cares, but guess what, it is the most beautiful sparkly twinkling piece of magic, embedded on a band that arches up, latticed like a bridge and trimmed with bunches of more diamonds, teeny tiny. I think I'm saying, "Oh my god oh my god," and just trying to get my head together and also *not* trying to get my head together because I understand this is one of those singular moments in life and I want to draw it out and sit in it, this timeless space, for as long as possible. And we kiss and I tell them how much I love them and then they ask, "So, you'll marry me?" in this voice like they *really don't know,* like they're *worried,* which is the most insane thing ever, even more insane then waking up to a diamond ring, and I say, "Oh my god, *of course* I'll marry you," and we make out some more, and I'm happy, I'm crying because it means my 40 milligrams of Citalopram aren't killing my feelings, and because crying while being proposed to is something women tend to do, and I like these occasional affirmations that I am normal. "Of *course* I'll marry you," I tell them, and then everything is a blur of crazy feelings and love and kisses and crying.

2013

ONE OUT OF FOUR; OR, DISAPPOINTMENT

1.

DIRTY GAY MAN-JUICE

It's time for our psychological screening with Dr. Posh. She looks like a middle-aged lady with some lesbian leanings and a head full of wild curls. She wears round glasses and has a copy of *The Lesbian Parenting Book* displayed face-out on her bookshelf.

Orson and I hold hands nervously through the interview. I worry that Dr. Posh will be discouraging or condescending or fear-mongering. That she's going to make Orson feel like an egg donor and me like I'm just a surrogate with no right to our baby. In general, we both fear a vaguely soul-crushing and anti-gay bad time. But mostly it's fine.

The doctor asks us about our history together. I begin telling her how I started inseminating on my own, with Quentin, and she interrupts me.

"Your time together," she says.

"I'm telling you about our time together," I say, and swiftly bring Orson into the story. That's the only hiccup. From there we talk about our relationship with Quentin, what we know about him, the conversations we've had. We learn that the paperwork they require Quentin to sign adequately removes his rights to his sperm and its offspring, so we don't really need to seek out a lawyer. She asks if Quentin has told his parents.

"No." We shake our heads. "He might at some point, but he doesn't have plans to."

"I'm going to advise him to tell them sooner rather than later," Dr. Posh says. "Usually the news is taken better if it's received at the start of the process."

I guess it's the psychiatrist's job to advise what's best for the emotional well-being of all involved, but as none of us—Orson, me, Quentin—really wants to accept that these biological grandparents are involved, none of us wants to think too much about their emotional well-being. I just know that if and when these folks learn about our kid, we'll deal with it. And my optimistic nature can imagine a million ways that having that extra set of grandparents could be a blessing.

Dr. Posh tells us it sounds like we're both on the same page and are communicating really well. She asks us to have Quentin make his appointment with her—we needed to have ours before he could have his. And she bids us adieu.

"We aced it!" Orson says inside the elevator, giving me a high five.

"It wasn't a test!" I giggle, because it sure felt like one.

"We aced it!" Orson repeats. They will repeat this throughout the day, administering high fives as needed.

I have to fill out waiver paperwork for the clinic that affirms I know that my sperm donor engages in SEX WITH MEN and *still* I'm allowing his dirty gay man-juice to impregnate me. This makes me so mad.

I have coffee with my friend Isis, who has a kid. She talks about how straight and white and middle-class the whole baby world is, even in the freethinking East Bay, where she lives. Isis has a man, but she's not white and she's not middle-class and she doesn't have a very heterosexual worldview, despite the man. She complains about how her prenatal yoga class refers to everyone's partners as "husbands." It makes me wonder, actually, what I'm going to call Orson once we're married. I rather like *husband,* frankly, even if it might make me invisible as a queer if they're not around and I'm all, *My husband this, my husband that.* But one of the really good things to come out of having been with a trans man for a while is having to let go of what the world thinks of you. Saying goodbye to the fantasy that it could ever understand you properly in the first place. That lesson coincided with getting sober, where I learned the phrase "What other people think of you is none of your business," a life-saving sentence if I've ever heard one. So I guess I don't care if the word *husband* as it leaves my lips conjures up a vision other than Orson. Who could imagine Orson anyway? I don't know if I've settled on the h-word, but it's certainly a more elegant, romantic choice than *spouse* or *partner.*

I tell Isis that I'm afraid of childbirth, and she tells me about how she was, too. "It's the kind of fear you can only deal with by going through it." More good advice. I just accept that I'm going to be super-duper scared, and decide to put off thinking about it till the contractions begin. Contractions, she says, feel like a cross between period cramps and gas pains.

How bad can it be?

After coffee with Isis, I go home and do a bunch of internet research, trying to find a therapist, because I'm guessing I'm going to need some support once I'm impregnated and off my meds. In the past, I was so broke and uninsured, I took what I could get. When I was twenty-one, that was an HMO woman I was allowed to see like three times, who ignored all the notes I had made on my intake form about having "disturbing sexual thoughts." All the masochistic fantasies I'd been having my whole life at the time seemed like a problem, mostly because I'd shared them with my boyfriend and they freaked him out. That, plus being on birth control pills that had me so hormonal I had to call in sick for a full week at a brand-new job because I couldn't stop crying, brought me to the HMO therapist. I don't remember her asking me anything pertinent. A few routine questions, and we were done. I wondered, if I was a man who had marked down I was having disturbing sexual thoughts, would the issue have been addressed? I'll never know, and I moved to San Francisco, where I swiftly met a landscape of sadomasochistic dykes and came to understand I was normal.

My next therapist, ten years later, was F-R-E-E *free*, because I'd told the free therapist office in San Francisco that I was going to hurt myself if they didn't find me someone to talk to, quick. I was at the first of many alcoholic bottoms, and hoped that with the help of a professional I could stop drinking without having to crawl on my belly to a 12-step meeting. Twelve-step meetings seemed like the worst thing that could possibly happen to a person, not to mention they were populated by people I had had drunken affairs with, people who had sobered up and now judged my drinking. I wouldn't give them the satisfaction of seeing me fall! Instead, I went weekly to this sort of lousy therapist who talked way too much about her eight-year-old daughter and confided to me that she, too, once thought that marriage was strictly for a man and a woman but she'd since loosened up. I cried in her office until I was desperate enough to hit a 12-step meeting, and then I really got better.

Three years later, I had another therapist, this one provided, on a sliding scale, by a New Age psychotherapy school in the city. I've gone to a couple of therapists who graduated from this place, and they are all specialists in the *Uh-huh . . . hmmm* school of talk therapy. Like, they just look at you while you ramble on and are all *Uh-huh . . . hmmmmm* about it. Even though I think this is total bullshit, I did love my therapist. Her name was Oona and I sought her out with Vito, when we were a couple and couldn't stop fighting. He insisted upon it after a scene on a beach in Florida, while visiting my mom, when I said, "All you do is spend my money and make me miserable!" I was proud of myself for speaking so boldly, but he was pissed and started calling potential therapists at the airport on the way home.

Oona had a sweet face and always looked really engaged, and when she spoke she had this darling voice that made me want to hug her to death. Even though Oona really did help me and Vito not fight quite as much, we still broke up, and I got to keep Oona. I went to her for a while, working through my pain at the break up and exulting in her affirmation that yes, I had been abandoned. I knew it! When I ceased caring and got happy again, I found myself trying to come up with problems to talk to Oona about, and it started feeling forced. She was a big fan of using therapy to talk about how rad your life is, too, but I got friends I can do that with. Friends who don't charge me thirty dollars an hour (cheap, right?). When Oona raised her rates to sixty dollars, I figured it was a sign from my higher power that I was done for a while.

Armed with this knowledge of therapists good and bad, I look at my computer screen, glowing with so many helpful-looking faces. I email the link to Tali and ask for her help. Tali is a therapy expert. She's written a bunch about her misadventures in sliding-scale therapy and has the initials of a particularly good therapist tattooed on her arm. I ask for her advice.

"*Don't pick one that looks like a slut,*" she tells me.

I roll my eyes at Tali. I would of course love a therapist with a slutty vibe. Such individuals are fonts of wisdom, the sort they don't teach in therapy school.

I pick a Russian therapist named Martina. I don't pick her *because* she was Russian, but I do hope that she possesses the tough-love, hard-assed depth that her countryfolk are famous for. One of her specialties is counseling people traumatized by war. You've got to have chops to do that.

But the thing is, just because a therapist is doing something doesn't mean they're doing it *well*. I sit across from Martina in a puffy white chair in a little box of a room. Though she wears the dowdy uniform of the therapist, the purse that was parked at the foot of her own puffy white chair was black leather and hung with gold hardware. I try not to stare at it. I instead stare into the face of my new therapist, her dark hair and her dark eyes.

I don't wait for Martina to ask me any questions. I jump right in: I'm an alcoholic, I'm sober, I'm queer, I'm trying to have a baby, I'm going to go off my meds, and I'm scared. When I'm off my meds, to the best of my memory, I become intensely dissatisfied with everything, am quick to get into a fight on the internet, need lots of rough sex, and cry a ton about my mom. Not looking forward to it.

Martina seems to think it is a good thing that pregnancy will be bumping me off my Citalopram.

"You don't want to have to take a pill every day for the rest of your life," she says, and my blood runs cold.

This is one of those weird things that people say about having to take a pill every day for the rest of your life: *You don't want to have to take a pill every day for the rest of your life.* I don't get it. What's the big deal? Taking a pill every day takes approximately one nanosecond. Gulp, it's gone. I guess I do have to walk down to Walgreens and pick up my prescription each month, but who cares? I have to do that if I want a bag of Jelly Bellys and a box of Tampons anyway. The underlying meaning is, *You don't want to be dependent on something for the rest of your life.* But I can promise you that being dependent on a little pill each day is waaaaaaaaaaay better than living with an anxiety condition that, left unmedicated, I try to medicate by making bad romantic choices, copious smoking, playing mad scientist with my diet, and shopping. One little pill a day that makes all of *that* go away, plus makes me stable enough to have a healthy relationship *and* pursue having a kid? I don't see the point of a discussion, even.

The unspoken sentiment here is that mental illness is not of the body; you just need an attitude adjustment. Because if you were struggling with any other sort of physical problem, no one would try to talk you out of the medication you need to feel better. As my mother says, "You'd take insulin if you were diabetic." She has always viewed the problems as similar, and now so do I. For whatever reason, I got some serious serotonin problems up in here.

I explain to Martina that as an alcoholic I already have to go to meetings all the time for the rest of my life, and that is much more of a pain in the ass than popping a pill. She seems delighted, genuinely illuminated, by this comparison. I tell her about the internet research I've done about people coming off my particular psych med, how miserable they reported feeling, how it worried me.

"Don't read things like that," Martina advises. "You will only upset yourself. It is important that you stay positive. You have a supportive relationship? That is something to focus on. What are your hobbies?"

Uh . . . did she just ask me what my *hobbies* are? I'm a writer—I don't have hobbies! I've monetized them—they're jobs! I don't even know how to answer this question. I try not to judge her. Okay. Maybe I do have a hobby. Reading? It's sort of work. I guess mindlessly flipping through fashion magazines and dog-earing pages depicting luxury items I'll never own is a sort of hobby.

What about cooking? Every day at around four P.M. I pack up work if I can. I clean the house and start cooking a meal for me and Orson. Sometimes it's something Spartan and wholesome from the *Clean Food* cookbook, sometimes it's something I pinned to my Pinterest dinner board. Orson's mom got us a subscription to the *Food Network Magazine,* and sometimes I'll cook from that. It took Orson a little while to get comfortable with me bringing them dinner every night while they sat on the couch in their sweats watching HGTV.

"I don't want you struggling over the stove for me," they said, concerned. "I don't want you to come to resent me." I had to convince them that I actually *love* getting to shut my computer and wrap my hands around some vegetables. It's the perfect way to transition out of the *I worked at home alone on a computer all day speaking to no one* spookiness and into something less heady, more grounded, ready to greet my businessman as they come in the door, hang their coat on a hook, and immediately inspect the dog for fleas. It's our little habit, and I really love it. I guess I do have a hobby, and it's cooking. Who knew? I learned something about myself in therapy after all.

I DECIDE TO STICK IT OUT WITH MARTINA, EVEN THOUGH SHE TAKES ANOTHER swipe at meds at the end of our session. "Your problems don't go away because you take a pill," she says, making it sound as if I'm mindlessly popping Klonopin. Actually, if the problem is your serotonin depletion, it actually *does* go away with the right medication. Grrrrr. Still, the thought of finding another therapist feels exhausting. What's to say the next one I pick will be any better?

While charting my and Orson's menstrual cycles for Stella the fertility nurse, I realize we both had PMS all weekend. That's why we had what I am now calling the Chuppah Fight Saturday night! The fight was basically like this:

Me: Do you want to have a chuppah at our wedding?

Orson: I don't know, I have to think about it.

Me: We've thought about it too long. Rhonda is going to do our flowers and needs to know what we're going to do with the stage area. Can we just commit right now, yes or no, to the chuppah?

Orson (picking up phone): How do you spell *chuppah*?

Me: I don't know, you're the Jew.

I am inordinately frustrated that Orson can't say yea or nay on the chuppah—the wedding canopy used in traditional Jewish weddings. Brenda and Finn had one at their wedding last summer, and it was beautiful. Plus, it symbolizes an open home, and I think if we get married beneath one it will be a good omen, or something that will at least mean we should host more parties.

Orson responds to my weird frustration with understandable coldness. I get it together and apologize for being such a bitch, go into the kitchen and do the dishes while silently crying. When I'm done, I come back to the couch and try cuddling up to Orson with hormonal desperation, anxious to make the coldness go away. I'm like one of those giant, fluffy cats who goes right up to the most allergic person in the room and jumps on their lap.

Anyway, it was just PMS! It's hard to track my hormones with my new birth control regimen; I just take active pills, no placebos, so I don't get a period, but I believe there is a mood-altering fluctuation there.

"I hope it was a happy household," Stella the fertility nurse laughs nervously when I exclaim my PMS revelation to her. Later, when I tell Orson, they declare that such hormonal influence makes the chuppah fight "not count." I couldn't agree more. PMS fights aren't real fights. Plus, we didn't yell, so it couldn't have been a fight, right? I kind of don't know if Orson and I either never fight or if our fights are these brief, tense moments that blow over too quickly to really register as *fights*. That we have both been in relationships where there were FIGHTS (ring that word in flashing lights, please) makes us more confused. Maybe we never fight, or maybe we fight really well. Maybe we're so conflict averse we just push the bad feelings aside, to accumulate into a pile destined to avalanche on us eight years hence? Time will surely tell.

Stella registers Orson and I for our IVF injection class. I realize that it falls during my mom's visit. She'll have to come with us! I actually think she'll like it—as a nurse herself, she'll feel like she's on stable ground. She'll be able to somewhat participate in the whole process, rendering it less mysterious. I wish Orson's mom could come, too! Take Your Moms to the Fertility Clinic Day.

Stella emails me my calendar and has me open it up on my computer while I'm on the phone with her. The calendars are a LOT. There's one for me and one for Orson, single sheets of paper that list all the meds we take each day, when to up the dosage, the adhering and removing of patches, phone calls to be made to nurses, blood draws at the clinic—it goes on and on, every day a jumble of tasks. The more there is, the more there is to screw up, I think. But people do this! People with fewer brain cells, less competence, less overall togetherness manage to do this, right? I guess it's *possible* that in the history of IVF, Orson and I are actually the dopiest, least together couple to ever load a syringe of Follistim, but the chances are certainly low. It's probably pathetic that I take comfort in this, but I do.

Stella is rattling off a bunch of drugs, all with creepy drug-names, like euphemisms for something sinister. Follistim and Medrol and Vivelle and Lupron and Menopur. Progesterone and Valium, too, but I know those guys. I ask Stella about side effects without even knowing which drug I'm asking about. How about *all* of them?

Hot flashes, breast tenderness, headaches. "It's going to be worse for your partner. They're going to have a lot of weight gain and mood swings." When Orson gets home from work that night, I have so much to tell them.

"Stella told me you'll have weight gain and mood swings," I report. "And that you're a candidate to stimulate a *lot* of follicles!"

I think this is good news, and it is, but it inspires in Orson a paranoid fantasy. "What if I make so many," they ask, "and they sell some of them? I wouldn't even know!" They chew their lip. "Should we ask them? Should we ask them if they ever take our eggs and do anything with them?"

"Should we ask them if they plan on raping us while we're under, as well?" I ask. "Because all of that is totally illegal."

"Don't be fresh." I love how Orson uses the word *fresh*. The only other people who use it in such a way, to connote brattiness, are, like, my mother. But I can see that Orson is actually worried, and maybe annoyed at me for making fun of their fears.

"I'm sorry," I say. "I'm not trying to be fresh, just funny. I mean, it would be so illegal for them to do anything with our eggs. I don't think we need to be concerned about that." I worry so little and Orson worries so much that we sometimes clunk against each other.

"You don't know what people do," they say ominously. But I'm pretty sure the clinic won't be selling our eggs on the black market. And if they do, I'll never know about it, so who cares. Unless I find out about it years later and then sue them for a million fucking dollars, in which case—awesome. Actually, the best thing that could happen to us financially is that the clinic steals some of Orson's primo eggs.

I call my mom and tell her everything. Now that I have the calendar, I can say that we'll be getting that embryo up in me at the beginning of July. I do the astrological math.

"We're going to have a fucking Aries," I say, so shocked and distressed that I use the f-word while on the phone with my very own mother. My mother cracks up.

"Aries are very generous and friendly," she says. "They're leaders. They're good with science."

Everything she says is true. I may know a larger-than-average number of self-centered, narcissistic Aries drug addicts, but I happen to know a larger-than-average number of self-centered, narcissistic drug addicts, period. I console myself with the good, even great Aries that I know: my friend Weezie, one of my favorite people. My ex Lindsey, who is super smart and together. The teen I mentor. And . . . I'm done. The faces of spoiled rotten Aries who live off the kindness of strangers bob in my mind like an Aries Chamber of Horrors. Oh, well. I've learned my lesson about astrological signs I supposedly don't click with. After a traumatic relationship with a Virgo, I swore them off for the rest of my life, only to find that date after date had a Virgo moon, a Virgo rising. And now Orson. A Virgo with a Virgo rising, and my most compatible partner yet. So what do I know? Baby Aries (well, that would be *baby* squared, wouldn't it?), bring it on.

When I hang up with Mom, I go back to Orson, and we review the calendars. Orson is breathing in such a way that I know their heart is probably fluttering and their pulse is surely racing. They turn to me. "We are ready for this," they affirm. "We are so ready for this."

"We are!" I concur as they grab their phone and start googling the side effects of every medication.

"Vivelle? What is Vivelle?"

"It's estrogen," I say. "But wouldn't it be a great name for a girl? Vivelle Bitman?" We've decided that we're all going to have Orson's last name. I'll keep writing under Tea, but that's never been my legal name. My real last name is my stepfather's, not even my biological father's. And I really don't want either of those guys' names. Orson is attached to their last name. When I think of taking their name, it's like their name is a big cozy sweater giving my name a cuddle. It's romantic and I love it.

I do sort of think Vivelle would be a pretty name if it wasn't already the brand name for a synthetic hormone. I also am really feeling the name Maple.

"No way," Orson says. "Hard no."

"Why not?" I ask. "Think about it. Maple. A little girl named Maple."

"Nope. I don't even like maple, we don't even eat maple."

"Yes, we do. All the time. There was maple syrup in our salad dressing tonight. Basically, whenever I cook out of that *Clean Food* cookbook, you're eating maple. But never mind." Orson is a California kid, born and raised in Sacramento. They can't relate to maple. I drop it before they counter by suggesting we name our son Tamari.

I tell Orson, as we begin our fertility med–induced descent into madness, that I really, really, *really* need them to tell me when they're stressing out or worrying about anything. Often, if Orson is dealing with stress, the way they cope is by not talking about it. This is anathema to me, totally against my self-help-y, therapized way of dealing with things, and it also triggers a deep fear I have of not knowing what is going on with my person and with my relationship. I beg Orson to always tell me everything, and they promise to always let me in, even though it is in their Virgo nature to crawl inside themself when things get hard. This night, our conversation deepens until we both share our most profound fears and tell intense family stories. I cry a little, but we feel super close.

"Is this what people mean when they talk about 'opening up'?" Orson asks, totally serious with their wide blue eyes. I start cracking up. Sometimes Orson is like an alien. A cute, innocent alien.

"Yes," I tell them. "This would be a good example of 'opening up.'"

The next day, while walking Rodney to the park, I find a book on the sidewalk—*The Secret Life of the Unborn Child*. I once would have scornfully disregarded such a thing as probable anti-choice paraphernalia, but now I am delighted by the find and feel that the Street Gods are smiling down on me and blessing my procreation attempts. I can't wait to learn about an unborn baby's secret life! I bring it home, even though I don't really bring things home from the street since Orson moved in, as they insist that everything on the street has been peed on by a dog. Now that I spend part of each day taking a dog to pee around the street, I see what a good point they have. Still, I smelled the book before I tossed it into my tote bag, and it smelled just fine.

Back at home, I place our fertility med order with a pharmacy in Encino. Of all the creepy drugs we'll be taking, Medrol creeps me out the most. It "quiets" the immune system. Euphemisms are generally creepy, and the way the clinic uses the word *quiet* whenever they are trying to chemically dismantle a vital physical system leaves a bad taste in my mouth. My guess is that some tech writer agonized over a word that would not leave women feeling totally freaked out at the thought of shutting down their defense against illness. *Shhh, hush now, you noisy immune system! Quiet down!* The thing is, my immune system might see the embryo as an invading monster and tear it out. So I do need to quiet it the fuck down.

I order progesterone and some Valium, which will be taken before the embryo transfer. By then, I believe I will have earned a freelapse.

Insurance covers one single box of the estrogen patch Vivelle every twenty-eight days, but I will be consuming four boxes of the estrogen patches in as many days. Four times as much estrogen as what it is normally used for, to replace the lost hormone in a woman's body. Should I be worried about cancer or what? I try not to google. It's not like I'm going to stop this procedure if I learn something unnerving. Generally speaking, I have accepted that I live in the modern world. Not only can I not stop any of it, I am deeply a part of it. We're all going to Hell together, I just bought my ticket early.

When I learn how much my meds cost, my heart actually lifts: $582.57. Why, that's barely more than the Helmut Lang dress I bought on sale to wear to my book party! Then the pharmacist gives me Orson's total. None of Orson's meds are covered by insurance, not a one: $3,492.90. I leave my body long enough to lose the thread of the conversation I'm having with the pharmacy and make it awkward. They're asking me for payment. OH! Of course. Doing fast, anxious math in my head, I give her my debit card. I have a late payment to the IRS due right now. I have money coming to me from a book I sold, it's just not here yet. In 12-step, we call this sort of dilemma a *luxury problem*. As the pharmacy woman reads the numbers on my card back to me, I repeat the little money mantra I got from my time in recovery: I HAVE A TRUST FUND FROM GOD.

This always calms me down. It totally shifts the way I think about my bank account. It doesn't matter if I think there's not enough in there, or if I'm happy with the amount but then scared to spend any, scared to watch the number tick down. It's actually *not* my money. It's god's money! She's letting me have it to do all the things on this earth she wants me to do. She'll make sure I have enough. And if it turns out I don't have enough? It means my god didn't actually want me to do that thing, anyway.

The pharmacy calls me back to tell me my card isn't going through. I call my hippie eco-bank and they inform me that I can't put transactions more than $1,500 on my debit card. Goddamn it. I remember I recently paid off a credit card. I grab the card and call the pharmacy, have them put that $1,500 max on my debit and do the rest on the credit card.

I MEET A WRITER FRIEND FOR DINNER THAT NIGHT, AND I AM LITERALLY SHOCKED to see her arms, which are covered in bruises. Serious bruises running livid from the straps of her tank top down to her wrists.

"I'm okay," she says with a wry smile, before I can even ask. I must have looked horrified, or she must be used to her friends having similar responses.

"Are they—happy bruises?" I ask weakly. I, too, enjoy getting romantically smacked around, and never want to yuck anyone's yum, but these bruises are a LOT. I didn't know my friend was so hard-core!

Well, she's not. She is part of a rare demographic of menopause-aged women who, rather than their estrogen petering out, actually get *more* estrogen as they age. She also recently had a blood clot, and the hospital sent her home with some kind of medicine that gave her a terrifyingly heavy period. When she returned to the hospital, they sent her home with another drug, to stop her from menstruating. *That* drug had the side effect of seizing all the muscles in her arms. She couldn't move them and suffered from intense muscle cramps. The bruises are from the extreme massaging and physical therapy she was enduring to get motion back.

"Oh my god!" I cry, aghast at her terrible story, sort of speechless. "What is the drug they gave you?"

"It's called Lupron," she says.

"Lupron?" I repeat dumbly.

"Yes, Lupron."

Not to make my friend's trauma *all about me,* but I just spent five hundred bucks on my own personal supply of Lupron.

"I'm supposed to be starting that drug next week," I tell my friend. "For IVF."

"Oh." She nods. "They must be trying to simulate menopause in you?"

"They're 'quieting my ovaries,'" I tell her. "So I don't get my period while they're manipulating my cycle for the embryo transfer."

"I bet they didn't tell you about the side effects." My friend laughs ruefully.

Egads, no. But I suppose when the meds arrive, they will arrive with unreadable scrolls of warnings that I will promptly throw in the trash. I think about how, if you think about the possible consequences of *anything,* you'd never get out of bed in the morning, right? And even staying in bed, well, think of all the consequences *that* could engender—bed sores! Atrophied muscles! Bed head! Of course we can't think about life in a way that prevents us from living it. And I can't think about the deeply artificial means it's going to take me to get pregnant if I do want to someday feel a little person jostling around inside of me.

2.

KNOWN EGG DONOR

I just don't think I'll have too bad a time giving myself progesterone shots after being in a relationship for years with Vito, a
trans guy whose testosterone I would inject into his derriere.
There really isn't a difference—his were for testosterone, mine will be
for progesterone, but the needles and the injection sites are the same.

The day the drugs are scheduled to arrive, I have to stay at
home to receive them, as some need to go right into the freezer. By
the time my friend Bananas comes over to kill the time, the package has already arrived. Orson's Follistim, the drug that will make
their ovaries produce a bazillion eggs, is in the fridge, but everything else is scattered all over the living room floor. I pulled all of
my vintage Pyrex containers out of the kitchen cabinets and am
trying to store the abundance of syringes and needles and alcohol
wipes in a classy and organized manner.

"Wow." Bananas takes in the scene. "It's like creepy baby
Christmas in here." Rodney gets involved, clambering over purple
boxes of Vivelle and green and white boxes of Menopur.

"Get off your brother." Bananas swoops down and plucks him off the meds. "When you get abandoned after this baby is born, I'll take you."

I make a mental note to never forget that Bananas has said this. On the one hand, Rodney is such a deep, serious part of our family, I can't imagine him not being around. On the other hand, there is the way he barks and barks and barks. What will that be like when we are beyond sleep deprived and just need the thing to quiet down and snooze for a minute? Will the baby wake up and sob? Will I sob? Will Orson?

What about walking Rodney every day? Can I handle a dog who pulls at his leash and does everything he can to eat every bit of shit—dog, human—in his path, while carrying or pushing a kid? What if I have a C-section? How long will it be before I can take him on his walks?

Sometimes I enjoy the way Rodney gives me a reason to leave the house each day. With Rodney I *have* to go to the park. But what will it feel like when there's a baby to be tending to? I can't imagine any of it, the unforeseen myriad of ways my life will change.

I wonder how serious Bananas is about taking Rodney if shit gets too hard, though I can't imagine ever agreeing to say goodbye to our good bad dog. And if I feel that way, Orson must feel that way times a million.

That night, it's time to start the drugs. I watch a video about how to give myself the Lupron shot, and it is truly no big whoop. The needle is super tiny and comes already attached to the syringe. The shot goes into my belly—anywhere below my belly button, beneath the "smile" made by the crease above my pooch. I take a pinch of skin and stick the needle in. Plunge the Lupron out. It takes less than a minute, and Orson looks at me like I'm a wizard. I do like feeling capable, and I'm relieved that this particular med is not so stressful.

I set up a calendar for coming off my psych meds. I know I

don't have to quit the Citalopram this soon, but I hate having this big change hanging over my head. Plus, as I begin to add all these creepy chemicals to my body, it feels good to be taking one out.

I run my detox plan past my sister, who had to come off meds to have her own kids. She thinks that if I stick to that schedule, I shouldn't feel any of the weird side effects people report when they quit cold turkey—flashes of light in their heads, nausea. I feel proud that I have finally figured it out and oddly psyched to embark upon this new chapter of the baby adventure.

An email comes in from the finance lady at the clinic. Her emails all come stamped with quotes from Joel Osteen and Margaret Thatcher, and so I hate her. The missive reads:

Hi Michelle,
Your nurse informed me you are anticipating an IVF cycle
using known egg and sperm donor. Please understand the
estimate is based on the protocol established by your M.D. and
is subject to change.

I type back to her:

Hello! Thank you for the information. The "known egg donor"
is actually my partner. Is there a way to better word these /
address them to us as a couple? Thank you!

It is hard to refrain from asking her to please omit the optimistic quotes from fascists from the tail of her emails, but I do, because I am keeping things PROFESSIONAL. It can feel really great to spin off and scream at a person—and I do—but I am often haunted by a certain feeling in the wake of it, a particular emotional hangover that signals I have surrendered my dignity. These emails with the clinic are like a training ground for me.

My calm falls away, however, when I see the attachment that came with the email: the bill for our test-tube baby. It's going to be more money than I've ever spent on anything. And even though Orson is quite gainfully employed and has heroically offered to take on most if not all of the baby payment, I'm trembling. Their money is my money and my money is their money and all of it is our money, and I'm suddenly scared of the great big chomp our unborn baby is about to take out of it.

The grand total is $14,000, plus another $700. I'd thought it was going to be $25,000!

I'm almost gleeful, as if we've actually won money. Orson is in an even more delusional state, having thought the bill was going to be for something like $30,000 or $40,000. We're flushed and grinning, our hearts racing like we just dodged a bullet. This is all so ridiculous; we've been delivered a rather large bill. But we've psyched ourselves into a state of crazed gratitude. A $14,000 bill is, like, nothing when you thought you'd be hit with a $40,000 one! Plus, I just sold my very first book to a mainstream publisher, earning my very first mainstream paycheck in two decades of publishing! The cash could not be coming at a better time.

We show up at the clinic for a meeting with Dr. Waller, who is talking to us about egg quality and marathons. "We're looking for the best, highest quality embryo, that's what we'll transfer. And some of the eggs will look good when we harvest them, but they won't make it to implantation. You know, I run ten miles a day, and I tried to run a marathon and I just couldn't do it. Some eggs are like that. Lots of great, functional people can't run a marathon. And some great eggs won't make that three-to-five-day wait." He looks at us, makes sure we're taking in all of this info. "We're going to implant one single embryo, because what you want is a healthy singleton. And that first implantation has a fifty-eight to eighty-eight percent success rate."

Whoa. Those odds are GOOD. I'm giddy, like someone just handed me a $14,000 bill all over again!

"Is the sperm source here?" Dr. Waller asks his computer, typing and frowning. Orson is watching him frown.

"Is everything okay?" Orson asks.

"Oh yeah," Dr. Waller says. "Just making sure you're listed here as the partner."

Orson and I exchange *Can you believe this goddamn place?* looks, and then Dr. Waller turns back to us and lets us go. We're done. For that five-minute check-in we're charged $111 back at reception.

"What are we even paying for?" Orson hisses, outraged.

"Who knows." I shrug. I hand my debit card to the fuchsia-haired lady behind the counter, and Orson makes a fuss.

"I wanted to get it," they protest.

"Don't worry," I say. "There will be *lots* of opportunities for you to pay." The fuchsia haired lady laughs along with us.

"Let me ask you," she interjects. "Did those tattoos hurt?"

"Yes," I said. "Yes, they did. Every single one of them." They hurt so bad that every time I get one, I wonder what the fuck I am doing. Why am I doing this to myself? But I am now too heavily tattooed not to continue to tattoo myself heavily. To be perfectly honest, every mother's warning has proven to be true, although it took about an extra decade to develop. I did not regret my tattoos at thirty, as many an elderly woman had predicted I would, but at forty. At forty I would like to have none of my tattoos, save the hearts I have on my knuckles. Maybe there's a rogue pokey heart I would keep, that's about it.

"I want to get one on my foot," the fuchsia-haired lady, whose name is Roya, tells me.

"You should do it," I tell her.

"Not if it hurts," she says, wincing.

"It just hurts in the moment," I tell her. "And then you have it forever."

3.

QUIET OVARIES

My mom is in town. She gets to finally meet Orson, whom she has only thus far spoken to on the phone, when they called to ask for my hand in marriage, a charmingly old-fashioned gesture totally on brand for Orson and their old-timey temperament. She is also in town for our injection workshop at the fertility clinic. I'm really glad we have the opportunity to show her where we've been going. She'll be able to see firsthand how sweet the clinic is, with its artful ceramic vegetable tiles lining the entry and the big landscaped courtyard.

The nurse who leads the workshop sort of resembles Sandra Bullock. Nurse Bullock explains the uses of the various medications, using the euphemism "quiet" again—the Lupron is to "quiet" our ovaries, the Medrol to "quiet" our immune systems. She brandishes a syringe: "This is an insulin syringe, short needle. You use this with the Lupron." Someone asks about side effects. "Maybe you'll get night sweats—who knows?" I'm actually prone to night sweats—my mother has been telling me I'm perimenopausal for like ten years now—but I haven't experienced anything so far.

"Throw that bad boy in the sharps container," Nurse Bullock says of the Lupron needle, and moves onto Ganirelix, one of the medicines Orson will be on to help their body create one million eggs. We learn that the terrifyingly long needle in our meds pack is a mixing needle, not a shooting needle, thank Goddess. We use it to draw up sterile water from one little vial and then inject it into the vial containing the medicine, which is a powder. Once it's liquefied, you draw it up into the syringe and swap out the needle for one that is considerably less horrific. Orson will shoot the Ganirelix into their belly.

I actually get a little bit confused during the powder-mixing part, but Orson assures me that they've got it down, so I don't worry about it. Nurse Bullock is talking about how the Ganirelix makes the ovaries swell. "You can sometimes feel them on the outside of the body," she says, and I throw up in my mouth a little. No, I don't. But, like, my soul does. Beside me, Orson shudders. It's all deeply gruesome.

Nurse Bullock then busts out a new euphemism: "selective reduction." It means having an abortion, in the case of having popped too many eggs into the uterus and, surprise, they all implant. Maybe this is more of a concern for people who aren't doing IVF but are using drugs that make you ovulate more than one egg. From what I've seen, the clinic is pretty intense about not transferring more than one egg during IVF, not unless there have been a few failed rounds and shit needs to be ramped up. She quickly moves on to cover ectopic pregnancy, when the egg swims back up the fallopian tube and begins to grow there, putting everyone's life at risk.

"Every week we see someone with an ectopic pregnancy," Nurse Bullock pronounces. There's something new to worry about. She tells us to watch for a "severe, one-sided pain" and, also, "don't go camping in Yosemite." Ectopic pregnancy is the reason you have to stay local for the two weeks following a positive pregnancy test. She ends this list of possible horrors with tales of ovarian torsion, when the ovary twists around itself, cutting off its blood supply. "It's very, very rare," she reassures us. "If you think you're having ovarian torsion, you're not."

Nurse Bullock moves on to Novarel, the brand name of the "trigger shot" that needs to be administered at the EXACT TIME the nurse tells us, thus triggering the ovaries to release all those millions of eggs. She drives the importance of the well-timed shot home by sharing the tale of a woman who did her trigger shot a half hour early. "By the time we got her into the retrieval room, her eggs were gone," she says darkly, and Orson and I trade *DAMN!* looks with each other. One woman nervously asks if it would be appropriate to carry the shot with her if she's not sure where she'll be on the day she's to shoot it.

"You can bring your hCG shot with you," the nurse nods. HCG, the trigger shot, is human chorionic gonadotropin, a hormone. "You and your partner can slip into a bathroom together and do it. Slip out after ten minutes, tussle your hair"—she gives us a saucy wink—"and be on your way." I shoot Orson and my mom a look. Who *is* this woman? Orson returns my facial sentiment, while my mother seems thoroughly entertained.

"Now, progesterone," the nurse continues, taking us from Orson's meds over to mine, "is administered with a one-and-a-half-inch needle that can go down to the muscle in your butt."

"Bummer," Orson says, looking at me tenderly. You can tell who in the room is on this protocol by the looks of terror on their faces.

"Progesterone isn't the unhappy hormone, but it does slow everything down," she continues. "You can expect constipation. It slows your G.I. tract down."

Nurse Bullock moves onto the men. She tells them it's not necessary for them to hoard their sperm in the days leading up to their procedures. "You don't have to save up for a couple weeks, because then your sperm is going to look like this." She crosses her eyes, sticks her tongue out and makes her arms all crooked and droopy. Okay, maybe I love Nurse Bullock. At the very least, she has found a way to make this presentation entertaining for herself, which I admire. She speaks to the men about the rooms where they'll "make their deposit": "Nobody's knocking on the door saying 'hurry up.' There's a lot of material, and you can bring your own material— nobody's going to laugh."

Once the men have been assured that no one will be laughing at their pornography choices, Nurse Bullock moves on to the egg retrieval. It takes only ten to twenty minutes, and is done with a sort of vaginal ultrasound wand that has a needle affixed to it. The wand gently probes into each follicle, aspirates the eggs out, and then the eggs get handed over to the embryologists. Then she moves back to the progesterone shots.

"I'm not gonna lie," she tells us. "I've had them. It was the most painful place I've ever gotten a shot." Orson, who has organized the contents of their baggie into a meticulous order in front of them, lifts up a very long needle. "This one goes in your ass," they say. I wonder if I can get them to do a pervy doctor role-play with me when we do it. Every night. For two and a half months.

A big bag of chocolate candy gets passed around. Class dismissed. My mother grabs a small handful and slides it into her purse. This is a family tradition. Her own mother was famous for stealing handfuls of creamers and sugar packets from diners. Her purse always had a tiny glass jar of jam inside it, a packet of maple syrup. When something free is set out, you take it. And then you take some more. Napkins, pencils. It's why I have been known to swipe a handful of tongue depressors from a doctor's office if I'm left alone too long. A compulsion and an inheritance. I collect my fake meds and sweep them into my own purse, glad my mom—who has viewed the workshop as a sort of cultural outing—stole some candy so I don't have to.

4.

LESS OF A CRAZY BITCH

May I outline some of the highlights of the weeks that followed?

Meeting Nurse Stella and discovering she is smoking hot: She has long, messy dark hair and turquoise chandelier earrings and generally looks like she should be modeling Pendleton clothing on a rust-colored cliff in Santa Fe. After the endless injections, we meet in her office to fill out a bunch of paperwork, including one form that asks us what we want the hospital to do with Orson's eggs should we die or break up. Well, we hadn't talked about this! The part about if we die is a no-brainer. If Orson dies, those eggs go to me, and I will spend the rest of my life giving birth to *all* of them, a Quiverfull of gaybies with Orson's elven features. But if we break up? Well, first, *it's not going to happen*. Orson and I are never going to break up; we're getting *married*. But unfortunately, so many other millions of couples have broken up—couples who at some point swore they'd never—that no one is going to believe us. So they make us fill out this stupid paperwork.

"Well, if we break up, I guess I sure don't want your eggs," I say glumly. Even having to consider this is hurting my feelings.

"Well, I guess I would want them." Orson shrugs uneasily, as confused as I am. "I mean . . . they're my eggs."

I see where they're coming from. Orson is reckoning with a scenario in which I've either heartlessly dumped them or done something unforgivable, thereby forcing them away from me. Of course they'll take their eggs with them when they go! They'll be taking their West Elm dresser as well, I suppose! Still, I feel like these are *our* eggs. I think that if we were to break up, they should be destroyed. But the whole thing is too foolish to get into, because we're *not* breaking up. So I sign off on the eggs going to Orson in the event that I am love-drugged without my consent and then placed in close proximity to, oh, Léa Seydoux or Ryan Gosling, who have also been love-drugged without their consent, and we put the moves on each other, and then Orson leaves me. Except I don't actually think Orson would leave me under these circumstances. But they're the only circumstance under which I can imagine cheating on Orson, so whatever. ONWARD!

Firing my therapist: Remember my dismissive Russian therapist? Dumped her. Came off meds and started shooting progesterone and LOST MY MIND. Like, crying all the time. Feeling like I should totally dismantle and throw the literary nonprofit I and others have spent ten years lovingly building into the garbage. Canceling writing classes and literary events because I just can't stop sobbing long enough to leave the house. I make an appointment with my new, elusive general practitioner, Dr. Louboutin, who confirms that there is *nothing* safe I can take to be less of a crazy bitch while undergoing IVF. No SSRIs, no herbs, nothing. She hands me some printouts listing various therapists, and I start going to a new one, Kenneth. Kenneth is older and sober and gay, all of which rule, but after a couple months visiting with him, I adjust to life on progesterone and off Celexa and don't have much to say. I find myself obsessing over how bummed I am that my stepfather was a Peeping Tom and how my mother stayed with him anyways, but this drama is over twenty years old, and I'm sick of talking about it. Does it make me feel bad? Yes, forever. I think Buddhist acceptance is more helpful than therapeutic rehashes at this point. And Buddhism is free. I fire Kenneth.

Orson getting harvested: This happens over gay pride weekend, which is extra proud this year given the good news around Prop 8 and DOMA. Our marriage will be *legal!* Now I won't have to legally adopt my fucking baby when I give birth to it someday, Goddess willing. After hanging out at the Dyke March, we run home and give Orson their trigger shot at exactly 8:15 at night. The next morning it's Gay Day, and we're in the hospital bright and early, in a room that looks out onto this hill where a bunch of gays created a big pink triangle. If I get pregnant from *any* of the eggs we get today, the conception day will be Gay Day, because the first thing they do when they grab Orson's gay eggs is douse them with Quentin's gay sperm and get them growing! I can't help but feel that this is auspicious.

When I meet back up with Orson after their brief procedure, they are all doped up and goofy and possibly happier than they've ever been. The number ten is written on their hand in Sharpie—it's how many eggs were harvested. They won't all make it to transfer, but it's a good number to work with. Super high on whatever they're pumped full of, Orson is insisting on thanking everyone who operated on them for their service. Even wasted, they are unerringly polite. Apparently, they were already buzzed when asked to state what they were there for, and they replied, "To get the golden egg." Our friend Lowell picks us up, greeting Orson with "You are the Eggman!"

Getting impregnated: I love being on the pills, even though the next day I crash and sob. But for the time I'm high, it's nice. The transfer is quick and painless, and the lighting is super groovy. The only snag is when the doctor doing the job—it's not Dr. Waller—asks us if we'd like one or two eggs transferred. What? Dude, I'm HIGH. Don't ask me to make a life-changing decision when I'm on pills! Plus, I didn't think we had a say. Dr. Waller said we were going with one, and that was that. We stick with the plan. Later, when we tell Dr. Waller about this, he seems miffed and makes a note on his computer.

Not getting pregnant: I gave myself the afternoon to cry about it. Orson and I console ourselves with not having to raise an Aries, and we meet with Dr. Waller to make a game plan for Take Two. This time around he wants me to stuff two Viagra suppositories up my hoo-ha each night. Apparently, the boner-maker has had great off-label success beefing up the uterine lining. We don't know if my uterine lining is why that last little zygote didn't attach, but why not cover all bases? He puts me on a regimen of aspirin as well, to thin out my blood, and it's back to shooting progesterone in my ass again. And again, it makes me feel fucking insane and tragic. We transfer another egg.

Getting pregnant: When Stella calls to tell me I'm pregnant, I'm on my way to a nearby crêperie for brunch. Before she calls, I just *know* I'm not pregnant, much to the dismay of my mother, who had a dream that I was and now believes it's true. My plan, after getting my not-impregnated state confirmed, is to drink a goblet of Colon Cleanse, because I have not shat in what seems like years, and then perhaps get a shot of Botox before our wedding. Why not? I got Botox a couple years ago and I freaking loved it. My forehead was lovely, and I didn't look at all frozen, just relaxed. It's too expensive to keep up with, but if a wedding isn't cause for cosmetic injections, then what is?

But when Stella calls, it's to tell me that I'm pregnant. This body of mine, that I've worried just wouldn't be a hospitable place for a baby to grow, is growing a baby. I start crying there on the street. "I just didn't think I was," I tell her.

"But why?" she asks, as if it was a given that I'd get pregnant. I can hear her smiling through the phone.

"I—I don't know," I stammer. "I just . . . haven't ever been pregnant before." I lean against an apartment building, just around the corner from the hustle and bustle of lower Haight Street. Dudes clatter by on skateboards, women walk dogs and drink coffee, giant orange city buses lumber to the curb, burp out some passengers, and roar on up the street. Life is totally normal, but not for me. I rub my teary cheeks with the sleeve of my sweater. Truthfully, it's not just that I haven't been pregnant before. It's that all through this process, months that surged into years, I never fully believed that I could be. And now I am. And life seems incredibly benevolent and magic.

Stella informs me that my hormone numbers are double what they should be, which makes her confident that it's not just a chemical pregnancy but the real deal. When I go in for another blood draw two days later, my numbers are again double what was expected. We go in for an ultrasound, and the nurse practitioner points to a tiny grain of rice on the screen. "There it is." She picks up a teeny-tiny heartbeat, but it's still early. When we return in a couple weeks, we can *see* the heartbeat. It flickers inside the embryo like a strobe light. "You're done here," the NP says happily. "Now that you're pregnant, we don't need to see you anymore. Find yourself an obstetrician. And congratulations."

Getting into the *New York Times*: I had submitted our engagement announcement to the *NYT*'s Vows section, just to be a queer and bougie bitch about it. And we got in! Not only that, a video journalist who makes little movies about future newlyweds likes our Getting Pregz story and is flying out to San Francisco to make a short about us. She's even going to accompany us to our first meeting with our new OB. "You really want the media there at your first ultrasound?" the timid media relations woman asks nervously. It's not our first ultrasound! It's our third, and we've *seen* the heartbeat. It's cool, man! The video journalist is cool, too. In her cat's-eye glasses and Converse sneakers, she's like someone I'd hang out with, and I feel totally fine about her being in the room when the OB slides her finger up my butt during the exam. What can I say? I'm a free spirit.

Our OB, Dr. Joan, is gray-haired and red-faced, Irish and portly, and I daresay a lesbian, though we can't be sure. She asks Orson if they'd like to take those pills that help you lactate so they can breastfeed the baby, too, and Orson goes white and shakes their head. The doctor laughs. "I've never seen a lesbian partner say yes," she says. We try to look at the baby on the ultrasound, which is not as high-tech as the ones at the IVF clinic, but we can't. "Twenty percent of women we can't pick up at this stage," she says. "It's nothing to be worried about." Okay, cool, then I won't worry. We hoped to get a shot of it for the video, but the video journalist asks if we'll take some footage at our next appointment and send it to her. Our next appointment, as it turns out, is the day before our wedding. Which is rad, because both our moms will be in town and can come see it, too.

Our next appointment. Orson gets nervous before all these appointments, but I don't. It just doesn't occur to me that anything will go wrong. It does occur to Dr. Joan. When once again she can't see anything, she's quick to get real about it. "You should prepare yourself for bad news," she says solemnly. "There is a chance that everything is okay, but we really should be able to see something right now." Our mothers look worried. They're both Scorpios, both prone to worst-case-scenario thinking. Additionally, my mother's nurse brain is brimming with all the things that can go wrong with a pregnancy. But me, I have the dopey good attitude of someone in serious denial. We're sent down the hall to a better ultrasound machine, and the woman rubs jelly over my stomach and presses down. She presses and presses and presses, then looks at me. "I'm so sorry," she says.

Orson and I hug each other and cry while Dr. Joan goes back into the exam room to break the news to our mothers. I can't stop crying, and daub at my eyes with a wadded-up napkin. I go outside and call Madeline and cry. I send text messages to everyone I told I was pregnant, asking them to please tell everyone *they* told I was pregnant that I'm not pregnant anymore. Friends call, but I don't want to talk to anyone. I can't believe we're getting married tomorrow, and everyone will be feeling sorry for me, and I'll be still looking totally pregnant. I'll have this sad little thing inside me, a little sack of cells that stopped growing two weeks ago, at eight weeks. I run a chance of miscarrying at my wedding—and yes, I'm wearing white!—so I'll have to pack my purse with pads. If I don't miscarry, I'll have to have an abortion. Too weird. Too awful.

Would you like people at the wedding to mention this or would you rather they didn't? Rhonda thoughtfully texts. It's exhausting to consider. *I don't know*, I text back.

Because it is the day before our freaking wedding, there is no time to collapse into the tears I would have if life was normal. Our families are in town, friends have come from all over. Orson has their hair appointment, and I have to get a mani-pedi. The only thing worse than this happening before such a special day would be the tragedy of it being visible from an uncharacteristically shabby appearance. Tomorrow's photos are going to be with us forever. After resting with a progesterone tablet in my vagina to stave off miscarriage, it's time to get up and go to our rehearsal dinner, to make it through the pizza party without having a meltdown.

OUR WEDDING

We'd been so looking forward to it, crafting our perfect day alongside our efforts to get pregnant, and it was unbelievable, as October bled into November, that we'd succeeded in both. We'd found the perfect venue, a vintage, wooden events hall on Market Street, darkly romantic with its beams and balconies. We'd gotten our favorite soul food restaurant to cater it, serving a fleet of pies in lieu of a wedding cake. Our sisters would be our maid of honor and best man, and my niece and nephew would toddle down the aisle, sprinkling flower petals and bearing rings. Rhonda did our flowers, and Tali would officiate, joining us in our commitment under a chuppah, which Orson did eventually fetch for us. More than being a nod to the groom's mostly ignored Jewish heritage, it's a beautiful, floral addition to the stage where we'd be married. I'd managed to find an empire-waist wedding dress to accommodate the possible size my belly could be come our November ceremony. At the last moment, my hairdresser volunteered to come and wind my hair into a braided crown, which I decorated with "something borrowed" hair jewelry from my sister. Everything looked beautiful, including us. But inside, we were crumbling.

We were getting married under the sign of Scorpio, one of the more intense signs of the zodiac. I'd hoped our marriage would be infused with the passionate and capable aspects of the sign, but as Orson and I huddled together in a private chamber at the back of the hall, awaiting our cue to walk down the aisle together, I feared the sign's association with death had marked the day, and I feared it would leave an imprint on our marriage as well. Before I could articulate anything, we heard the procession begin and, facing each other, grabbed hands and burst through the wooden doors and out into our ceremony.

I was so worried that the miscarriage news would turn our wedding into a sad event, but, as I watched rows of our guests turn to receive us, I felt amazed by the radiant love and support blazing from them. Tali's thoughtfully crafted sermon spoke to queer rights, and how could it not? When Orson first proposed to me, this ceremony would not have been legally recognized. Tali, and most of my friends present, came of age thinking we could never have such things as weddings, and so we spat upon them, snubbed the institution as it snubbed us, not necessarily asking ourselves if it was what we really thought or if we were just protecting ourselves. For lots of people, it was complicated. Tali burst into tears speaking about it, the ambivalence and joy, the hard past of queer people and the precariousness of this new moment we stood on the very tip of.

Then it was time for our vows. Orson began theirs by saying my name in this lovely, clear way and looking at me so intensely, it made me dizzy. Our first promise was to caretake and nurture our love, so that it continued to grow and thrive. We promised to pet each other's head, to snug and be snugged, to respect each other's autonomy.

I had a hard time getting Orson's ring over their knuckle, and they had to sort of do it, but they wouldn't let me take my hand away; they wrapped their fingers around mine and we jammed that thing on together. And then we were married. We went and hid out in that back chamber together and kissed and caught our breath before going out to greet all the people who had come to cheer us. And they really did cheer! When we walked down the aisle, holding hands, everyone stood up and started screaming. I hadn't expected that. Orson did a big fist pump. They hadn't planned to do it, it's just how they naturally express joy.

After our wedding was over, and everyone was gone, we stood outside the venue, me barefoot, no longer able to walk in my Lanvin pumps. We took a cab to our room at the Fairmont. The Fairmont is the fanciest hotel in the city, and it seemed like we should spend our wedding night someplace really fantastical, someplace that we'd never been and would never be again. I got the room half price on Ootels.com, the bargain hotel website for people who don't know how to spell *Hotel*. It was perfect to lie around in fluffy hotel robes and go through our presents, but it would have been nice if I wasn't miscarrying and we could have engaged in traditional wedding-night activities, like sex. It was Saturday night. My abortion was still five days away.

Why did it take me almost a week to get an abortion? Well, my schedule was a little intense that week, but also the Women's Options Center is only open *two days a week*. How in the world can that be enough to accommodate all the ladies in San Francisco who need abortions? It made me think of the book *Generation Roe,* which talks about how scarce abortion services are across the United State because of the pressure put on providers, be it from the legislature or from death threats.

Though it is ridiculous that providing a basic medical service to women in this day and age should be seen as noble and radical, I do think the work the people at Women's Options are doing is both noble and radical, and I salute them. That said, I did not need the intake nurse, Dolores, to talk to me like I was child who'd become separated from her mommy in a big department store. Her walking-on-eggshells voice, every sentence ending in a gentle up-tone, made me want to die. I'm sure they've had to deal with women freaking out in every which way, so maybe this tone and timbre is practiced and often useful, but it made me feel like an infant or an imbecile. I was so happy when Dolores left and one of the doctors came in and just talked like a normal person. I still felt compassion and sympathy from the doctor; you don't have to speak in a baby voice to convey such things. After that doctor left, another doctor came in to introduce herself. She was midway between Dolores and the normal doctor in terms of talking to me like I was having a mental breakdown. Which I was not. I was not having a mental breakdown. I wanted this clot of cells taken out of me so I could go on with my life. Once I learned it didn't have a heartbeat and had stopped developing weeks before, I'd ceased thinking of it as my future child who would grow up and do wonderful things, and had begun regarding it as a strange, gelatinous bit of sea life that had washed up on the shores of my uterus.

After Dolores went over my paperwork, with that voice that was so gentle it was like a horrible, faint tickle all over my *soul*, I was allowed to pop some Vicodin and ibuprofen. Orson and I waited around for the pills to kick in; then one of the doctors came in to explain that the Novocain-like stuff they use to numb my cervix might make me feel dizzy or nauseous or give me a metallic taste in my mouth. The upshot of this is that it's really strong and I should not feel any pain at all.

After a couple hours, it was finally time for me to don my ass-less smock and climb onto the table. I was super doped up at this point, and when they started numbing my cervix, I felt a wave of intense, psychedelic dizziness. For a moment, it felt like the room and everyone in it—Orson and Dolores and the two doctors—were very, very far away. Orson said I turned super, spooky white. But then the sensation faded, and it was happening.

My abortion team's plan for the procedure was apparently to distract me as much as possible from what was going on. Dolores and Dr. Number Two kept up a steady stream of inane chatter, getting us talking about our dog, the postwedding brunch at the Fairmont, where we were going on our honeymoon. The pressure to engage was sort of exhausting. I was so doped up, I didn't want to talk. If I made any sort of noise someone—or all of them—would quickly ask if I was in pain. No, no, no pain. But I could feel a terrible *tugging* deep inside, a yanking. If there was a lull in the conversation, Dr. Number Two would look at us wildly and start yakking. I was glad when it was over and I could be alone in the room with Orson, lying there high until it was time to go home.

5.

GOOD NEWS AND BAD

Right after my D and C procedure and right before Orson and I leave for our honeymoon, I have an appointment with Dr. Laser. She's a psychiatrist Dr. Joan, the OB, thought I should see back when I was pregnant; she thought it would be a good idea to get a postpartum plan together in the event I slide into madness once the baby was on my teat and all my hormones had leached away. After the ultrasounds revealed that the baby had stopped developing, Dr. Joan still thought it would be smart to talk to Dr. Laser. Why not? I figured. It has been a season of hiring and firing therapists; might as well bring a psychiatrist into the mix. As it was, I felt a bit numb. There was a bubble of loss around me, moving with me when I moved, but I was too distracted to pay it much mind. We were coming down from the wedding, looking at pictures, fielding congratulations on the internet and in real life. We were stocking up on sunscreen and making lists of last-minute items we'd need for our honeymoon. The D and C, though distressing in its way, melted into just another procedure during a season of them. And Dr. Laser was, perhaps, just another specialist whose office I'd enter and exit.

But Dr. Laser is sort of foxy, somewhere in her thirties, with long cherry-red hair and tall black boots. I'm both comforted by and distraught at her apparent coolness—it makes me feel like she'll understand me, which wakes me up a little, but it also makes me want to impress her, which is embarrassing. Dr. Laser keeps a pretty solid therapy poker face, asking me a series of questions that prompts me to reveal exactly how fucked up I've been, in how many different manners, for how long. I detail my family history of alcoholism and some other stunning achievements. Yes, I have had some dalliances with eating disorders—OCD, too! Awesome. Depression, anxiety. There was that time in my late teens when I couldn't stop crying. There's that whole deal with my stepfather. I started out on Lexapro, switched to Celexa, and then hopped to Citalopram. Now I'm off everything, detoxing, no doubt, from the pregnancy hormones, natural and synthetic, that have flooded my body for the past few months.

It feels so lousy to have to detail the vagaries of your inherited mental health. I mean, if I'm hanging out with my similarly banged-up friends, making dark jokes and cracking up at our shared gallows humor, it's awesome. At a 12-step meeting, such revelations seem almost sacred, meaningful, helpful—and, again, absurdly funny. But sitting in a tiny office while a medical professional makes notes on a computer feels overwhelming.

Dr. Laser has good news and bad. From my history with hormones—getting PMS, having my birth control pill meltdown at eighteen, flipping out on my progesterone shots—I am likely to suffer postpartum depression after childbirth. The fact that she is even optimistic that I *could* become pregnant again is a shock, as it does not feel like a given to me right now. It feels like: Of course I miscarried. I totally would miscarry! My body can't create life!

Regardless, Orson doesn't like that postpartum projection one bit, but Orson is superstitious. They think that by saying some-thing like "You'll probably experience some postpartum depres-sion" dooms me to spending the first year of our offspring's life cutting myself in the bathroom. But I feel like we're just being real with each other, Dr. Laser and me. My sister suffered from post-partum, and so did my mother, and so did her mother. I feel very sensitive to the hormonal tides of my body. If we look at this thing honestly, we could get a plan together before I even have my next bun in the oven, which is what Dr. Laser would like to do.

The good news—remember, I told you there was good news in here—is that Dr. Laser thinks I take fabulously to antidepres-sants. Many people struggle to find a pill that's right for them, that doesn't make them feel worse or give them diarrhea, and then they have to figure out the dosage, often through some gnarly trial and error. Not me. I've hopped around a bunch of pills and have only had awesome responses. Because of this, she thinks I'd do well on Zoloft, which is the med that works best for mothers who need little helpers. Some women take Zoloft throughout their pregnancy or while nursing—only a negligible amount gets passed through the breast milk. None of that coming off serotonin that Dr. Moody Butch had mentioned what now feels like twenty years ago. At the very least, I can take Zoloft for postpartum, but Dr. Laser thinks I should try some now, so that we know for sure it sits well with me when I really need it.

I'm a little torn. Part of me would love to take the Zoloft right now. It would be really nice to be on meds again, feel that balanced ease, not worry that a scroll through my Facebook feed could leave me ensnared in a virtual slapfest with a virtual "friend." But then, the thought of having to titrate off it when I get pregnant again worries me. (BTW, I love the word *titrate*. It sounds so snappy and elegant, like a purposeful young lady clicking around in a smart pair of Kate Spades, holding a clipboard.) Am I just screwing myself up so hard coming on and off all these chemicals?

But what if this next round of IVF doesn't even get me pregnant? It would take another two months to try again, and that's like . . . three or four months I could have some chemical support. It seems risky to go without it.

I decide to try the Zoloft. My plan is to take it until I'm actually pregnant, and then titrate off the stuff. (Again, *titrate*, an Audrey Hepburn–esque woman walking down a very minimalist, white spiral staircase in a pair of kitten heels—are you with me?) If some women safely stay on the pills throughout their whole pregnancy, then surely it won't be very dangerous to have the stuff in my system for just a month or so.

I tell Dr. Laser to call the prescription in for me. Later, I toss it into my toiletry bag with the prenatal vitamins I have to keep taking even though the iron is *not* helping my constipation, as well as melatonin, some of my natural Swiss Kriss laxatives, and the ibuprofen I have to keep around in case the D and C cramping starts up again. And then, to top it off, I pack sunscreen and after-sun lotion and bathing suits and the new pieces I grabbed from the sale rack at Urban Outfitters that fit over my body, which still looks a little pregnant, though less so. It's time for our honeymoon.

6.

I AM HER MOTHER

When Orson and I booked our honeymoon, we hadn't even had our first embryo transfer yet. We did the math: if that initial zygote implanted and grew in my belly, then I'd be about five to six months pregnant come honeymoon time. Some women thrive beneath that onslaught of hormones and physical changes; some are miserable. We decided to take the gamble.

One thing Orson and I love is a beach vacation. So much of my travel is work-related that beach locales tend to be the only spots where I'm able to actually unwind and read for fun. Orson had gone to the Caribbean as a kid and loved it; they wanted to show me the rolling islands and bright blue waters. We checked a cruise line and found a ship going to the Caribbean a week after our wedding.

We were a little concerned about experiencing homophobia on the cruise. While we did get some stink-eye here and there, people were mostly friendly. They wanted to know if we were on our honeymoon. Uh, yeah, we would admit. This was a very chatty cruise.

I responded to our fellow cruisers warily. I have learned the hard way that most strangers will inevitably say something that totally offends me, and I wind up mad at myself for trusting humanity, while debating internally if it is worth it to get into a fight with the asshole or just abruptly ignore them. In this case, though, everyone was pretty harmless.

Orson and I spent a lot of time hiding out in our cabin, watching endless DVDs and eating endless room-service popcorn. We were exhausted from our wedding and from our miscarriage; for the first half of our vacation, I bled nonstop into fat maxi pads. We steered clear of everyone and created our own little world of two, and we did a good enough job enjoying our honeymoon in spite of our recent trauma *and* in spite of the people on the islands who repeatedly asked us if *I* was Orson's *mother.* Really? Their *mother?* I'm only eight years older than them! I would have to be at least fifty-two years old to be her mother, and that's if I had managed to give birth to her at the tender age of twelve. Do I really look fifty-two?

The first time it happened, it struck me as so comical, so absurd, that I nodded and said, "Yes, yes, I am their mother." However, confirming this woman's assumption only seemed to have confused her further. Now she seemed to not believe me. "*You* are *her* mother?" she demanded suspiciously. Perhaps she had known we were lezzies but felt she couldn't ask, so decided to ask if we were instead mother and daughter, in the hope that we'd correct her. But really—*mother?* Hadn't she heard of the classic "Are you two sisters?"

As funny as I thought it was, it really bothered Orson. When it happened again, in a shoe shop in St. Barts, they quickly snapped, "No, she's my wife!"

"Oh—wife," nodded the Italian boy selling us shoes, who looked to be about fifteen years old. I *had* been acting like a naggy mom, telling Orson exactly *why* the suede driving moccasins were such a good deal, insisting they get a pair, coaxing them away from the hardware and toward the tasseled style, then insisting upon which color was superior. I guess we were enacting a bit of a teenage-boy-shopping-with-mom dynamic. Still, if we're going to do mommy play, I want to be in on it, not have it projected onto me by strangers. We paid for Orson's driving moccasins and left.

Coming home from our honeymoon was bittersweet, as all ends of vacations are. We missed the luxury of getting to spend all day every day together. I missed the blue water and the rolling bumps of island dotting the horizon. But, ten days later, we were back in our San Francisco bubble. Home, sweet home.

WHEN I CAME BACK FROM MY HONEYMOON, EVERYONE I ENCOUNTERED HAD terrifying CONGRATULATIONS! for me. Terrifying because I didn't know if they were offering a congrats for my wedding or for my pregnancy, which was no more. I live my life on the internet, and in the wedding photos people were commenting on, I looked hella pregnant. Someone I'd never shared anything with posted on my Facebook wall about how excited she was to see my baby pictures. So, with every congratulations, I tensed up, not sure how to respond.

At my least graceful, I blurted, "I'm not pregnant!" leaving the kind congratulator to stutter and explain, "I meant about your marriage." So I started asking, "Oh, what for?" Which is probably totally weird coming from someone who just posted her wedding photos all over the internet, but I always have my reputation as a space cadet to fall back on. "Oh right—my wedding!!! Thank you!!!" After one woman whom I nervously snapped "I'm not pregnant!" at sent me a sweet message detailing her own experience with miscarriage, I started to calm down. Kind of. A little.

One thing I wanted to happen pronto was for my body to return to its prepregnancy state. Even though it was only all the progesterone shots and estrogen patches making me look pregnant, the fact was I *had* been pregnant, and I had looked pregnant, even if what everyone was seeing was just a few undigested burritos. If I thought it sucked to be mistaken for being pregnant when I was aspiring toward pregnancy, it super-duper-*uber* sucked to get mistaken for being pregnant after I'd miscarried.

I decided to try out the yoga studio around the corner from my new place. Yoga seemed like a gentle way to introduce some physical activity back into my life, and the side effects of calming my mind would be welcome. I put on a pair of pajamas (my workout clothing and sleepwear are interchangeable) and got there early enough to lay my mat out in a prime location on the floor.

It had been a very long while since my last yoga class, and even at my most ardent, I don't go regularly. Still, I'm usually able to keep up. Not this time. My body trembled and sweated. Normally I can barrel through a yoga class, but in this one, my failures way outnumbered the little moments of triumphs that made me feel strong. As I assumed each asana, my body felt totally foreign to me—lumpy and tight, weak and achy.

Giving myself permission to default to Child's Pose whenever the struggle became too stressful was a slippery slope. At one point, I started to cry. I'd fallen so out of touch with my body over these past months of on-again/off-again exercise. Enduring nightly shots of progesterone, feeling my body constipate and bloat, the weird food cravings and repulsions during my pregnancy—of *course* I was out of my body. It had become a sort of gnarly place to be.

Lying facedown on the floor in the yoga studio, hearing the motions of the people around me as they lifted and descended into their streams of poses, I was suddenly overcome with grief. I had hardly cried at all about my miscarriage—there had been no time. I hadn't *wanted* to cry, in fact. I'd wanted to exult in being married to Orson, in our love, to go on our honeymoon. So that's what happened, and now here was where I landed—back in my body, once again, but in a yoga studio lit by those horrible, tacky LED candles.

When I finally stood back up and resumed my attempts, the tears flowed, but in the dark no one could see.

I cried for my poor, sweet body, and all it had been through. Two rounds of awful Lupron and the anxiety and depression it engenders, without the help of my beloved antidepressants, not to mention coffee and orgasms, nature's psych meds. Two rounds of nightly progesterone shots to the ass, so that wide patches were dense with scar tissue and a strange mixture of numbness and pain. Two rounds of estrogen patches. A round of Viagra up my hooch. Ten weeks of pregnancy, with all the queasiness that accompanies it, evil smells jumping out at me from everywhere. An abortion, the gross, strong tugging, the crazy cervical anesthesia that made me pale and dizzy. The pads and pads of blood. Ugh. I sunk back down into Child's Pose and wept. It all crashed down on me, and my body felt very small, very fragile, and very beaten.

After a few days of stretching myself to the edge, I thought to myself: *Fuck yoga*. I turned to the only other physical activity option in my new hood—the motherfucking ocean. I bundled myself up in my warmest pajamas and stole one of Orson's beanies, plus their woolly gloves and the weird little jogger's fanny pack they have even though they don't jog or really indulge in any exercise whatsoever. I put on my sunglasses right as the sun was coming up and walked down to the dunes.

Just climbing over the dunes was a bit of a workout, leaving me winded. I set the timer on my cell phone for five minutes. My plan was to begin there, and each morning add an additional minute. I didn't really know what my goal was—like, how many minutes I planned to work my way up to. I knew that people ran for hours, which seemed terrifying to me. But then, not drinking for a year once seemed terrifying, too, though I hadn't had a drink in ten years and it was no big whoop. So anything was possible. But for now—five minutes.

I was gasping when it was over, gratitude at the timer's shrill beep coursing through my body. But the next morning, I was dying to do it again. An addict can get addicted to anything that pumps out those excellent happy brain chemicals, and I could feel the effect the running had on me. Bathing in the ocean's groovy negative ions *plus* the lovely Zoloft kicking in didn't hurt either.

The best thing about jogging on the beach was how not boring it was. How could you be bored at the ocean! The waves are magnificent and full of batshit crazy surfers riding the frothy curls in their alien suits. There are endangered little snowy plovers with the quickest skinny legs, and seagulls big as tomcats. Fishermen jam their poles into the sand and kick out into the water in their thigh-high waders. It's a whole, fantastic world, the ocean. I'd beachcomb the shore on the way back, collecting sand dollars and barnacles, and blend a kale smoothie when I got home. And after a while, I stopped looking like I was pregnant and was able to fit back into my black Rag & Bone jeans. And then it was time to try to get pregnant again.

7.

FOUR EGGS LEFT

Freshly back from our honeymoon, we reunite with Dr. Waller. He pauses briefly before moving to let us enter his office. "Bummer," he says soulfully. I appreciate both the brevity and the genuineness. It is indeed a bummer that our embryo stopped developing, when it had been looking so good. It is indeed a bummer that we're back at his office putting together Plan B. Or rather, Plan C.

"We were so close." He shakes his head regretfully while pulling files up on his computer. "Was there any diagnostic testing done?" He means, did we send the stuff dug out of me during the D and C to a lab to try to figure out what went awry? We did not. Per the advice of Dr. Joan, we declined, as she'd told us that such testing was expensive, insurance was unlikely to cover it, and if our plan was to go ahead with the next eggs in line anyway, it didn't really matter.

Dr. Waller tells us we have four eggs left in the freezer. He suggests transferring two into my uterus this time, and we agree.

If it means we wind up with a creepy set of twins who talk to each other in a secret twin language and prank us endlessly and love each other more than they will ever love us, their parents, then so be it. At least they'll always have each other. The more I think about it, the more I feel sort of excited at the thought of twins. It's the only shot we have at a larger family, as I am sure as fucking hell never going through this again. Maybe we'd adopt a sibling, down the road, but it's more likely that we'll have one spoiled rotten only child who thinks the world revolves around them. So a set of twins could be good.

Then I think about breast-feeding two squabbling babies, and having to maneuver them out of the house every day to walk the dog, and having to send them *both* to college. The gnarlyness of having two babies growing in my body and all the risks that go along with that. Now I feel nervous about two embryos being catapulted up my vag. I remind myself that Dr. Waller isn't transferring two to give us *twins;* he's implanting two because, odds are, one alone won't result in a baby for us.

After the meeting with Dr. Waller, I call the Encino pharmacy and order my next round of drugs. It's the same protocol as last time: birth control pills, Lupron shots, estrogen patches, progesterone shots, Viagra suppositories, Medrol, aspirin, and—hopefully, once pregnant—transitioning from progesterone shots to progesterone suppositories. It comes to one thousand dollars, and I know I'll need refills.

Starting the meds this time around feels different after the miscarriage. The novelty has worn off. Gone is the weird thrill that came from shooting myself in the stomach with a little needle. My trusting, giddy optimism is also gone. We now know from harsh experience that I can go through all of this and not get pregnant; we also know from experience that I can get pregnant and have it just stop. This time I'm just going through the motions, as if I have some sort of medical condition that requires me to give myself shots and pop these pills. It feels disconnected from our hopes of having a baby. It's just, like, what we *do*. We pinch the fat on my belly and stick a needle into it. Every single night.

After some weeks of ingesting the appropriate meds and sliding those crumbly bullets of Viagra up my snatch, the results are in: my uterine lining is measuring a whopping *nine* whatever-unit-of-measure-is-used-to-measure-uterine-lining. Last time it was six and a half; this time they were hoping for a seven. A nine is amazing! I imagine my uterus as a fluffy heaven of plush pillows and lush goose-down comforters, the sort of place you'd like to recline after indulging in some opium, the sort of place any embryo would *kill* to implant itself! We are sent to meet with Nurse Luz, who will prep us for the next stage.

Nurse Luz spreads out a bunch of paperwork on her desk, pointing to the row of dates at the end of January when a transfer would likely take place. The three possible dates were clustered around the new moon in Aquarius. How auspicious! My January horoscope had predicted something nice for me at the end of the month—not the thing itself, but the first step toward a long longed-for something. A new moon is always a great moment to initiate something, the start of a fresh cycle, so it was perfect for an embryo transfer.

My astro-obsession continues as I do some quick math and determine that the resulting baby would be a Scorpio. Or Scorpios. Scorpio twins! Holy shit! (An astrologer friend will later tell me, with a dismissive flip of his hand, "Don't worry, you'll never have Scorpio twins. One would eat the other in the womb.")

Orson and I are quite pleased at the possibility of a Scorpio child; both our moms and sisters are Scorpios, and some of my greatest friends (like Rhonda) are Scorpios.

It's probably our astrological destiny to continue the line of intense little power-mad creative geniuses. Bring it on!

As it happens, Nurse Luz is herself a Scorpio, and like many

Scorpios, beleaguered by an astrological reputation that pegs them all as psychopaths and nymphomaniacs. Which they very well might be. But they're also *capable* and *passionate!*

"Any sign can be messed up and crazy," I assure Nurse Luz. "Scorpios are just extroverts and popular, so they affect a lot more people when they're damaged. Cancers and Tauruses can be crazy, too. They just lock themselves in their homes and cut their arms and nobody knows what a mess they are." Nurse Luz really likes this. She offers to draw the circles on my butt with a Sharpie so I know just where to stick my progesterone shots, and I let her. It makes sense that, with our marriage a Scorpio, the fruit of our union would be that wild, impassioned star sign as well.

2014

INVASION OF THE
BODY SNATCHER; OR, JOY

1.

A BONA FIDE ZYGOTE

One month before our third-time's-a-charm embryo transfer, I get horribly sick. It goes on for about a month, morphing from a sore throat to a chest cold to what feels like a whooping cough. On the phone with a friend, my eye, which had been a little itchy, just starts *weeping*. Oh god, oh gross, this cannot be good, I tell myself. I call my GP, whom I can never get an appointment with, assure her that I have properly diagnosed myself with pinkeye, and beg her for an antibiotic. That night I am squeezing a medicinal gel into my eyes and stumbling blindly around my home, compulsively washing my hands. Orson trails behind me with a fistful of Lysol wipes.

I got the flu shot, for the very first time in my life, back when I was pregnant, so I know this ever-changing, epic illness is not the flu. The only bright side of it plaguing me from Christmas Day all the way up to our frozen embryo transfer on January twenty-eighth is that your body is actually more susceptible to getting pregz when your immune system is busted. My sister tells me that she was so sick when she got pregnant with her daughter, she and her husband almost didn't try that night. So I decide my lingering malaise is a good thing. This, plus the transfer date being the new moon *and* the date that Susan Miller predicted I would *plant the seed* for something I've been wanting for a long time (!!!), has me feeling pretty optimistic about this transfer.

On the drive to the transfer, I tell Orson about the family sicknesses that occur when you have kids, how the entire family—Mama, Baba, and whatever children are scurrying around—all get whacked with the same illness at the same time.

"What are we even doing?" they cry, suddenly desperate. "Should we just be traveling instead?"

"It's kind of too late for that," I say, popping my single prescribed Valium. Soon we're back in our scrubs, being led into the dimly lit room, where I climb onto a table and allow a kind gentleman to pass a couple of thawed embryos through my cervix. I have such sweet feelings about this room and this procedure. Maybe it's because I'm always pleasantly high on the first waves of Valium while I'm there, but they really know how to light the place, and everyone is so gentle and tender and full of well-wishes. And when I leave, I have—at least for the moment—a living embryo in my uterus. What's not to love?

On the way home, we make our customary stop at Bi-Rite Market, and Orson goes in to fetch me an ice cream cone while I wait in the car. Why do downers make ice cream taste so magnificent? At home, I lie on the couch and watch *Broad City* while Orson fixes dinner. I find myself wishing Orson would take a pill, too, so we could both lounge around on pills and cuddle.

"We'll never lie around on pills, having sex," I say mournfully to Orson as they bring me a bowl of soup.

"I think that's probably okay," they console me.

If we are to find ourselves legitimately knocked up from this transfer, Orson wants us to wait before we tell anyone. I have mixed feelings about this, but I'm high and was only just moping about not being able to have sex while freelapsing, so I don't trust my reactions, and let the suggestion marinate. After our miscarriage, it was a bummer to have to go back and tell everyone that the baby we'd gotten all excited about wasn't actually happening. It would be a lot less complicated to keep it to ourselves until we got the all-clear. Except you never get the all-clear. Something can always happen, and I am at this point the repository of enough worst-case-scenario pregnancy stories to know that we're not out of the woods until I'm holding a healthy newborn baby to my teat.

While the miscarriage sucked away a lot of my optimism, once the embryos are up in there, I get really excited again. I start calling them "The Twins" and texting double dancing girl emojis to friends who knew we'd gone in for another round. Orson asks me to stop. So I do. Then I start calling them my "Embabiez," having picked up that one while trolling some TTC message board. Orson also asks me to stop that. Like their request to keep the happenings in my uterus close to the chest, I understand why they don't like me talking about the little nubs like they are sure things, microscopic personalities jam-packed with cute, hanging on to my uterine wall like a couple of Sanrio characters. But that's how I feel about them! I am so happy that they are in me, and though I know that nothing might ever come of them, I just can't help but feel as if they are sweetly nesting inside me. But I don't want to make any potential harsh tokes any harsher for Orson, who has seemed to go full steam ahead with a self-protection regimen, so I stop calling them the Twins or the Embabiez. Except in texts to all my friends and in my head all the time.

NOT LONG AFTER THE TRANSFER, I'M DUE TO FLY TO THE EAST COAST FOR A couple nights, to lecture at an art school in New Hampshire, then to Santa Cruz for a conference on maternity. Who will give me my shot? The one I get in my ass, every single night, with a big freaking intramuscular needle? I tried giving it to myself once, back at the start of these shenanigans, when I was off my precious psychiatric medication, and had burst into tears. Since then, it has been on Orson. Now, not only do I have to find someone to shoot me up in New Hampshire and Santa Cruz, but Orson is leaving for a family get-together the night before I fly out, so I'll need someone to give me a shot right here in San Francisco.

This is immediately overwhelming. I turn to Sandwich, knowing that she is way too squeamish to deal with putting a needle into a friend's buttocks, but also knowing she is such a loyal friend that she'll possibly do it. In New Hampshire, the head of the English Department, who is bringing me out to speak to her classes, vaguely assures me we'll figure something out. In Santa Cruz, I hit up Quentin, as if he hasn't already done enough to try to get me pregnant. At the end of it all, I feel somewhat exhausted and that I am foisting something a tad too intimate onto friends and strangers. I cancel with everyone, even Sandwich. I'm going to have to learn to give myself my own goddamn injections, tears or no tears.

I call my ex Vito, who learned to give himself his own testosterone when the doctor at the trans youth clinic got sick of seeing his ass every other week. He learned to do it by bullying himself in the mirror: "You want to be a man, you little bitch? Do it. Do it." I take solace in knowing that my ex, who really *could* be a big baby about things, has mastered it. I try it on my own the night before Orson leaves town, so they can coach me. They redraw Nurse Luz's circles on my butt, and I step up to the mirror.

Taking a deep breath, I stretch the skin on my ass and sink the needle right into it. I am grateful I don't have to do it by myself all the time, like many people do; I know I'm not doing the best job of it, and I fear the lasting damage I could do to my ass. But for less than one week, me and my ass will manage. I kiss Orson goodbye, knowing that I have everything under control.

Sometimes when I am in an airport, I very badly want to eat McDonald's. I can get into an occasional Quarter Pounder with Cheese and a Supersize fries, which is what I eat at the Chicago O'Hare airport while waiting for my connecting flight to New Hampshire. I feel slightly bad about it only because I don't want to give my Embabiez the wrong idea, that if they implant in my uterus I'll punish them with a diet of pink-slime patties and sugar fries. But I justify it by thinking that, if my plane crashes and I die, I will be so mad at myself for not indulging my last earthly guilty pleasure.

A little bit after I eat my *fucking delicious* Quarter Pounder with Cheese, I have these little cramps in my abdomen. It could be my body smacking me for the abuse I just dealt it, or it could be . . . implantation cramping! Am I pregnant, or did I simply eat Mc-Donald's? How many women ask themselves this every day? To take my mind off it, I go forth in search of magazines and decide to buy a fancy chocolate bar while I'm at it. The woman rings me up, and it comes to a bazillion dollars.

"How much is the chocolate?" I ask.

"Four dollars," says the woman.

I am no stranger to four-dollar chocolate bars; I live in San Francisco. I am certain I have paid double that for some exquisite confection dotted with sea salt hand-harvested by French nuns on the coast of Normandy. I have the four dollars in my wallet, and it's not going to put me in the poorhouse to splurge on a sweet. But for some reason I just feel *irritated* that the chocolate bar is so much money, and I rebel against it and put it back. The woman watches me with a concerned face.

"You can just have it," she whispers. She makes a round motion over her stomach. "You're pregnant?" she says, and nods.

Normally I would jump at the chance to assist any minimum-wage worker in a bit of workplace sabotage, especially if it results in some free candy for me. But I'm so taken aback at the pregnancy comment that I'm flustered and confused. I pay for my magazine and leave without the chocolate, looking down at my belly as I walk back to my gate. I look pregnant *already?* I won't even be able to pee on a stick for a week and a half; my official blood test is a good two weeks away. I'm not quite as annoyed/despairing as I normally am, because by now I'm fairly used to it. At least, I console myself, I actually, truly, for real *might* be pregnant. Like, a day or two pregnant. Wearing a skintight dress with horizontal stripes isn't really helping. When I peek at myself in the bathroom mirror, I decide I easily look four months pregnant.

IN NEW HAMPSHIRE, I VISIT WITH SOME ENGLISH CLASSES, JUDGE A POETRY slam, and give a reading. After the events, the department chair takes me out to dinner, and I order a falafel plate that comes on a salad. I devour the falafel, but the salad is repulsive. I choke down a few leaves in a sad attempt to offset the effects of the airport Mc-Donald's.

"Is it not good?" the department chair asks with concern.

"No, it is," I tell her. "I just can't eat the salad for some reason."

The department chair is a mom, and she knows I may have one or two fertilized eggs hooking themselves to my uterine walls.

"You're pregnant!" she hisses.

"Do you think?" I gush. I remember that when I was pregnant last time, everything green was totally grotesque to me. I normally eat a lot of kale, broccoli, and spinach and string beans and bok choy. Now all I want to eat are baskets of deep-fried falafel and bags of Quarter Pounders with Cheese.

From New Hampshire, I fly to San Jose, where a car service takes me to Santa Cruz for the symposium on maternity.

"So," says the driver, making conversation on the way to the parking lot, "I see you'll have a nice surprise coming this spring." We both look at my belly.

Spring? Spring starts in *March*. It is *February*. Do I look *eight months pregnant?* Let's say he meant May. Do I look *six* months pregnant? Holy god. These progesterone shots—which, BTWs, I slid into my ass a bit crookedly but totally successfully while in New Hampshire—really *transform* a lady's body!

The driver is looking at me expectantly.

"We'll see," I say lightly and evasively.

IN MY HOTEL ROOM IN SANTA CRUZ I FIND BLOOD IN MY UNDERWEAR AND AM gripped with a weird, clashing emotion that is part excitement, part dread. It could totally be implantation bleeding. This is when it would happen, especially if those cramps *weren't* fast-food gas after all! It could also totally be, like, my period or something. It could be anything, it could be nothing. I find myself surging with hope, which some stern internal voice quickly scolds me for: *Don't get your hopes up. The higher they go, the harder they fall.*

Orson and I decided that we wouldn't use any home pregnancy tests this time around—we'd just wait for my blood test to give us the results. But upon returning to San Francisco from my travels, I decide against my own best interests and walk into a Walgreens to buy a box of pee tests.

"Look what I bought," I tell Orson when they get home from work that night. "I won't use it if you don't want me to."

"Well, why would we?" they ask.

"Because maybe it will tell us we're pregnant. If it says we're pregnant, we probably are. And if it's negative, we might be pregnant anyway."

"Well." Orson thinks it over. "We have to be ready to see a negative and not get upset."

"A negative isn't really a negative," I reason.

"Then why are we doing it?"

"I don't know," I respond. "I just want to *do* something. It really might tell us we're pregnant."

"Okay." Orson relents, with a smile cracking across their face.

The next morning, I face the box sitting on the back of the toilet. I haven't peed on a stick in so long. There is a familiar comfort in the routine of it, even though it has never given me the information I want. I uncap the stick and pee over the fibrous tip. I close my eyes and drift; I still have a lot of sleep in me.

Then I look at the pee stick.

It is positive. The unmistakable pink line deepens even as I watch it, mouth open. It gets pinker and pinker till it's pinker than the test line. My heart bobs in my chest, and I get a surge of chills that make my body wiggle in a silly dance. I take a breath. I shove down the excitement and walk lightly back into the bedroom, where Orson sleeps under blankets. I clutch the stick in my hand and burrow in next to them. I find their ear beneath the fold of a sheet.

"We're pregnant," I whisper into it.

When Orson is sleeping, their bones melt away, and they are just this floppy creature that flops around some but mostly lies very flat and still. When I whisper to them that we are pregnant, they roll over and envelop me in their floppy, boneless arms. It is like being embraced by a life-size stuffed animal.

"Where are your bones?" I ask them. "How do you get so floppy?"

"You have to do another test," they murmur in their floppy half-sleep. "We have to make sure."

"Okay, Flops," I promise. We doze for a bit in a dreamy way, and I am happy it is the weekend and neither of us has to go report to computers somewhere. We can just laze until someone—me or the dog—needs to pee.

After I pee on the second stick, I watch it turn palest pink, pale pink, faint pink, legitimately pink, dark pink, deep pink, hot pink. I bring both pee sticks back into the bed with me. Is that gross? I just peed on them. But they are magic wands now.

"Look," I say in a hushed voice to Orson. "We are so pregnant."

They hustle upward, their bones solidifying. "Oh my god," they say, the *d* in *god* getting stuck in their mouth.

"Oh my god!" I agree.

"Let's not tell anyone," they say. My blood test is midweek, but I feel pretty sure. Two BFPs in a row after POAS with FRER? (That's two Big Fat Positives after Peeing on a Stick with First Response Early Result brand pregnancy pee sticks, for those who don't troll TTC message boards.) I know that I'm at least very chemically pregnant. Whatever happens from this point, as we learned so recently, is up to the gods, but I know I'm pregnant, that the sticks are right. But if Orson wants to wait until we get the results of the blood (beta-hCG) tests, that's fine.

"We can tell our families," they say, and we immediately call our mothers and sisters.

"Tali and Bernadine count as family," they say, and I shoot off a text to Tali and Bernadine.

"You know," I say to Orson, "people know we did an egg transfer. If someone *asks* if I'm pregnant, someone who knows I had some fertilized eggs in me, can I be honest?"

"I guess," Orson says uneasily. I don't like making them uneasy, but I need to know what to do in this awkward situation, an awkward situation I know I'm going to be in soon. Like, that afternoon. More friends text asking if we're pregnant yet or what.

"Can I tell Joe Blow and Madame X we're pregnant?" I ask, looking down at my phone.

"Fine," Orson says, in a tone of voice that conveys it's actually not fine at all. I acquiesce and tell the incoming texters that we won't know until midweek. Which, if we'd followed the fertility clinic's advice and not done a home test, is when we'd know. We're totally not even *supposed* to *know* we're pregnant right now! But we do. And I want to tell everyone.

WE GET IN A MASSIVE FIGHT ON OUR WALK TO THE GROCERY STORE. WE MOSTLY only fight on special occasions. When something totally awesome happens, we have a big blowout. This is preferable to fighting on the daily, but frankly, totally awesome things happen to us all the time, and I wish we weren't cursed with this weird-ass pattern.

I feel oppressed by Orson's need to keep things quiet, to protect themself. I thought, if I *do* miscarry again, I don't want to carry it around like a big dark secret. Orson agrees, politically, that it is bad for women, the way everyone is so hush-hush about this common tragedy. But they still don't want everyone knowing their business. I don't know why I am possessed with such a desperate need to make sure the entire *world* knows *my* business, but I am, and I poke and needle at Orson's protective resolve until we are fighting in the street. As if we were in a movie, rain comes down all around us. Orson spins around and stomps home, while I collect myself and go into the grocery store to get food for dinner. I defiantly grab an expensive San Francisco health-food-store chocolate bar, planning to eat my feelings on the soggy walk home. I eat mouthful after mouthful of wet chocolate while the rain wears away at my paper grocery bags until they finally split just as I walk into the front yard, produce spilling all over the place, rolling up against the honest-to-god white picket fence that surrounds our home. I lift the wet groceries off the little patch of grass, the brick walkway that leads to the door. With dread in my belly, I let myself into the house.

Back in the house, we fight some more, going in circles, Orson defending their right to some privacy, me psychoanalyzing their need, deeming it "fear-based" and therefore unacceptable. I storm back out into the rain, thinking I'll punish all of us by walking along the ocean in a storm, after dark. By the time I get to the corner, I realize it is an exhausting exercise, and so I go home. I feel like a kid who's threatened to run away from home and instead sulks in the backyard for a half hour, then goes back inside to their stuffed animals.

Worse than fighting is being pregnant and fighting. My stomach feels deeply empty and hollow even though I've eaten a bunch of food, a sensation I remember from when I was pregnant last time. My hunger is located exactly in my stomach, a lonely place I can feel between the bottom of my ribs. I have no appetite, yet my stomach roars. I lie in bed and dab at my eyes with a lacy hankie. I'd accumulated a lovely collection of vintage lady's handkerchiefs back before I went on meds, when I cried all the time and thought I should at least inject some style into it, for my self-esteem. Now I have a cute little collection in my top drawer, mostly from a thrift store in Scotland.

Eventually, Orson and I stop fighting and go to sleep. And then we get over it, though I don't even remember how. Fighting is so stupid. Who cares if nobody knows I'm pregnant? They'll know soon enough, since I am somehow already showing.

The next day I get a call from the fertility clinic.

"I'm doing great," I gush to the nurse on the phone. "And I took a home pregnancy test and it said I'm pregnant. Two of them did."

"Well," the nurse says, with a tinge of warning to her voice. The clinic really doesn't like you taking the home pregnancy tests, because a false negative could cause a person to go off their hormones, sabotaging a pregnancy that might actually be viable.

"That's great," she says mildly. "We can be cautiously optimistic."

Cautiously optimistic? Cautious optimism was my state *before* the test. The whole reason you pee on a stick is to bump that cautious optimism up into *careful euphoria*. I try not to let the nurse's restraint bum me out too much, but I am surprised at the disappointment in my chest when I get off the phone.

The morning I get my beta-hCG test, I wake up in bed naked and covered in sweat, the sheets beneath me a shallow pool of wetness. I definitely had pajamas on when I went to sleep; I must have

ripped them off in my night-sweats frenzy. Even though the pajamas feel unbearable in the midst of a sweatfest, it's actually more
disgusting to be naked, because there's nothing to absorb the sweat
puddles and also I stick to the sheets. I'm a monster.

I take a train and then a bus into the Marina, getting off at the
stop near the Marc by Marc Jacobs store, walking up the hill to the
medical complex where Dr. Becky, my beloved gynecologist, has an
office. Our insurance won't cover anything fertility related, so my
fear is that if I get the beta-hCG test through the fertility clinic, I'll
have to pay for it. I make sure the results get faxed to the fertility
clinic stat.

In the late morning, while waiting for Nurse Angie to call, I
get a call from Dr. Becky, beloved gynecologist. The results have
hit her office first.

"You're pregnant!" she declares happily. Dr. Becky knows the
drama I've been through to get to this state, and now: a bona fide
zygote attached to my uterine walls, and growing!

"That's so great!" I gush to Dr. Becky. "Does that mean that
both the embryos attached? Am I having twins?"

"There's no way for me to tell," she says.

After we hang up, I sit, very still, at my kitchen table, thinking
about all the signs of pregnancy I'd experienced leading up to this
moment. The offer of free chocolate, the chauffeur's congratulations, the repulsive lettuce..I realize I'd *felt* it, I'd known I was pregnant, but I didn't dare say it, for fear that it was wishful thinking
and that I'd feel even worse when I was proven wrong, *again*. I lace
my fingers around my belly in that annoying way pregnant ladies
do. It's a pose I'll assume with increasing frequency in the coming
months, giving my baby—and my body—a hug. I was so proud of
this body, and all it had gone through. I imagine that it had been
studying, all these months, learning how a body becomes pregnant,
and it had cracked the code, it had figured it out, my body was

teachable, and together we'd taught it to become fertile, to grow an imperceptibly small swell of life within it.

TWO MORNINGS LATER, I'M UP AT SIX A.M. AND HEADED ACROSS THE CITY ON A series of trains and buses to get my second blood test. After my blood has been taken, I'm insanely hungry and walk down to a restaurant that makes great shakshuka. When the skillet is set steaming at my table, my stomach clenches. Isn't feta on the no-eat list for pregnant people? And the eggs aren't cooked through, they are perfectly, deliciously runny, and aren't runny eggs off-limits, too? And then there's the coffee. A latte. I promise myself I won't drink all of it, maybe just half, just enough to give me a little glow. As I dive into my skillet, I think about how I'm already a bad mother. I'm no different than any addict who thinks that whatever baby-ruining chemical she's ingesting is somehow no big whoop. What if this coffee provokes a miscarriage? What if I get *Listeria* or *Salmonella* from the totally scrumptious breakfast I can't stop inhaling? I am as powerless over my cravings as my mother—who was allotted six cigarettes a day *by her doctor* while she was pregnant with me—was over hers.

I feel like, if my mom smoked six cigarettes a day and—*Look!*— I turned out all right, then surely I can eat my shakshuka. This line of reasoning doesn't really make me feel better, though. Is this the sort of low-standards bartering I want to engage in as a pregnant person? I haven't figured any of this out by the time I clean my skillet, mopping up the tomato sauce with hunks of bread. I abandon my half-drunk latte.

Nurse Angie calls me right away. "I wanted to give you the good news first! I was ripped off last time!" It must be one of the better parts of Nurse Angie's job, telling the people who just mortgaged their home to get pregnant that a little test tube baby is growing inside them.

Nurse Angie tells me what I want to hear: that my hCG numbers have more than doubled since the test two days ago. This is excellent news: that little nub on my uterus is really growing!

"Do you think," I ask Nurse Angie, "that I could have twins? And that's why my numbers are so high?" I ask this question with both fear and excitement in my heart. Fear, because—let's face it—people who have twins are *fucked*. I know it's the happiest fucked state you'll ever be in and you wouldn't sell off one of them to the circus for all the dollar bills in the world, but still. You're sort of fucked.

"There's no way to know from the numbers," Nurse Angie says. "You'll just have to wait for your ultrasound." She goes through the list of foods I need to avoid, triggering my breakfast shame spiral all over again. But something she says snaps me out of it:

"Limit your caffeine intake to two hundred milligrams a day."

"So I can have coffee?" I practically scream into the phone.

"Oh, sure," she says casually. "You can have a cup of coffee."

"Exactly," I say, as if I'm somehow negotiating with her. "That's all I want, just one cup of coffee a day."

Nurse Angie laughs. "It's no problem, enjoy it."

Oh, you bet I will enjoy it. There will be no more weeklong meltdowns and losing of the mind this time around! I'm on Zoloft *and* I can drink coffee! I am going to be the happiest, least hormonal pregnant bitch in town!

2.

MAYBE A FAVA BEAN

Orson gets really excited when I get nauseous. My nausea isn't terrible—I'm not puking or bedridden from it. It's more like a constant, low-grade queasiness that I like to whine about. "I'm sorry, baby," Orson says with a big grin, and asks if they can fetch me anything.

I understand why Orson gets so gleeful about my sour stomach; pregnancy symptoms are a good thing. Even though I had nausea during my last pregnancy, and that didn't stop things from going awry, the fact is, being too grossed out by dog food to feed Rodney or being able to smell Rodney across the room even after he's had a bath are positives. Even as I complain about them, I'm happy about them, too. Now, if only my boobs would get bigger. I would like to have some pregnancy symptoms that are actually enjoyable.

No one is telling me I look "radiant" or like I'm "glowing," compliments I was collecting last time around, but I was always suspicious that said radiance could be traced back to the Burt's Bees Radiance Serum I was slathering onto my face every night, and, wouldn't you know it, since I've *run out* of this beauty potion, all radiance-related compliments have declined. Beauty products *do* work! But also, the miscarriage that followed that radiant moment of pregnancy may have people a tad inhibited to comment. Hard to say.

I'm anxious for our upcoming ultrasound, which will reveal if there are one or two little jerks gestating inside me. As the days tick on, my symptoms bloom. Leftovers are banished. The sight of a Pyrex full of something even as innocuous as a day-old bowl of beans and rice makes me gag. Everything gets tossed into the compost.

And finally: my boobs *are* getting bigger! I make Orson grab at them every day, not in a sexy way (like, no, really, it's not sexy), asking, "They're so big, right?????" while I flex my pectorals.

"Don't *do* that," they say, dropping the muscular thrust of my boob from their hand. "They're big enough without you doing that, it's just weird." I stop doing it, but there is something strangely satisfying about the little bit of oomph my boobs get when I flex. It's like they're my awesomely tough boob muscles.

Because I am not allowed to have any orgasms, lest the little zygote(s) are blown off my walls with the force of contractions, I am seriously sexually frustrated. This results in me having wild, perverted sex dreams practically every single night. They star everyone from skeezy old men to Nikki from *The Bachelor,* during this, the Juan Pablo season. Nikki is the one with the long bleachy hair who wore a slightly heavy-metal-looking gown and is a pediatric nurse. In my dream she's sort of butch, a combination of herself and Cara Delevingne. It's not a bad dream at all, but I do wish I could have an orgasm. Instead, I get hiccups. Did you know that hiccups are a pregnancy symptom? Pregnant people breathe faster because they need more air to accommodate how much more blood their bodies are producing, and this can cause hiccups. The wonders of the body!

It is my suspicion that every little weird, glitchy thing happening to my body is somehow related to being pregnant, and I don't seem to be incorrect. When my contact lenses suddenly feel strange on my eyes, I consult the interweb, and lo and behold, pregnancy changes *the shape of your eyes*. Wild! I guess it makes sense that something as monumental as *growing a person inside your body* would change your whole body and not just your uterus, but it's fascinating to learn how total the effects are.

While all of these wondrous things are happening to my bod, I'm a bit haunted by my hunch that IVF pregnancies have a higher incidence of stillbirths. Maybe it's because a stillbirth story just ran on my momming magazine, *Mutha,* a little website I started back when I was overwhelmed with the cheesy TTC message boards and was longing for the stories of parents I could relate to. It's low-key taken off, with compelling first-person stories of parenthood landing in my inbox every day. The stillbirth story felt intense to run, but it was absolutely the type of honest storytelling I craved, and if I was gauging our readers correctly, they wanted such raw reality as well. But the editor—me—wasn't thinking about the potential effects of the story on newly-pregnant-again-after-a-miscarriage me.

As if I was a glutton for anxiety, I then, after months of avoiding it, finally cracked open the memoir *Ghostbelly,* in which Elizabeth Heineman recounts her relationship with her own stillborn baby. Recently, a friend experienced a stillbirth, and my heart felt permanently sagged with sadness at what she had to go through. I remind myself that none of these people—my writer, Elizabeth Heineman, my friend—had utilized assisted reproductive technology (ART) in their pregnancies, but then I begin reading Miriam Zoll's *Cracked Open,* a scathing critique of the Fertility Industrial Complex that questions if any of these reproductive technologies work at all. It is a bad time for me to begin my own personal Baby Bummer Book Club, but I forge ahead, nerding out on my own anxieties.

FINALLY, THE DAY OF OUR ULTRASOUND COMES. I'M IN THE STIRRUPS WATCHING our friendly Nurse Practitioner Jennifer roll a supersized condom thing onto the Wand. Orson looks at me and grins, hopeful and nervous and supportive and slightly comic all at once. Jennifer slides the beast up my vag and—presto—there, nestled against my uterine wall, is a lima bean. Maybe a fava bean. Maybe even a peanut, still in its shell. I note with both relief and disappointment that there is only one little bean in my belly, and Jennifer, sliding the wand around inside me, confirms. We have a singleton. A totally healthy singleton who is developing ahead of schedule.

Jennifer knows about our recent miscarriage and encourages us to feel happy and optimistic about this news. "You have a one-in-four chance of miscarrying, every woman does," she explains. "And you just got your one out of four over with. There's no reason to believe this pregnancy won't be a great, healthy one." She's happy for us, and I'm eager to believe her. Even though we started this round of IVF with a new hesitation, even gloom, my pessimism burned away after the transfer, and I've felt positive and excited in spite of myself. In spite of the specter of that last miscarriage, in spite of traumatic memoirs and googled medical studies, I'm giddy with this bean in my belly, and it seems dumb to try to talk myself out of it by imagining worst-case scenarios. I decide to be happy and enjoy being pregnant.

It's not until we're back in the car, eating the ice cream cones we always get, that I realize I forgot to ask Jennifer if I can stop having sex dreams about contestants on *The Bachelor* and have a real-life orgasm. Goddammit! Orson takes their eyes from the road and gives me a pleading look.

"Why not just forget it for a little longer?" they beg, making me feel like a frenzied sex addict. "We have our whole life to have orgasms. Let's just wait a little longer. Please?" *Easy for them to say,* the cynical among you may be thinking, but let me tell you that

Orson has also pledged no orgasms for the duration of my abstinence, wanting us to suffer together. I really admire this, though I in no way require it, and encourage them to, you know, take care of their own business; there's no reason for us *both* to be sexually frustrated. But Orson is a team player. We keep our hands off each other, and don't make out, as kissing swiftly leads to other things. Their vibrator collects dust in their bedside table and mine collects dust bunnies under the bed. We haven't even had our baby yet, and our sex life is already compromised.

3.

PICKLE JUICE

Having had it with my sexual frustration and the attendant dirty dreams my psyche was screening for me each night, I call the nurses' station at the fertility clinic and bluntly ask if I am now allowed to have orgasms.

"Yes, of course," says the nurse. "You could have been having them for the past two weeks."

Hear that, Orson? *The past two weeks!* Weeks that I've spent all shot up with hormones, enduring sex dreams about Charles Bukowski and Coco Rocha (separately). I begin masturbating immediately, now knowing that it is *perfectly safe* for me to be using my Hitachi Magic Wand, the lawn mower of sex toys.

Meanwhile, my body is growing. While I expected my midsection to rise up with the growth of my *bébé*, I didn't know I would no longer be able to get my thrifted Ferragamo boots over my calves. I wake in the morning to find that my labia have bloomed during the night and now spill out from the crotch of my underwear.

Really? I'm gaining pregnancy weight in my *vagina?* I turn back to the internet, wondering—not for the first time—how pregnant women got through the day back when they couldn't just pick up a magic gadget and have the answer to their latest neuroses flashed at them in a millisecond. Up pops a blog post titled "My Swollen Vagina and Other Things Nobody Told Me About Pregnancy." I don't even have to read the essay; just the title is enough to reassure me. Orson takes me to Target and I purchased some underwear roomy enough to contain my phat new labez, wondering all the while what will be the next area of my body to do something astounding, what new baby-propelled mutation awaits me.

ONE AFTERNOON, AS I AM BEGINNING TO PREPARE DINNER FOR ORSON AND ME, I become gripped—gripped!—by a craving. A pickle craving. Pickles have always been a favorite food, and I can crave them even when not pregnant. But now that I *am* pregnant, what once tasted wicked good now tastes frigging *marvelous*. I'm finding that this is the thing with pregnancy cravings. It's not so much that you are overcome with a panting, desperate need for some food you'd never normally eat. It's more like, the stuff you generally enjoy takes on this whole new dimension of deliciousness. I'm so into pickles right now, I'm even hankering for those sweet bread-and-butter pickles, which I normally don't care for. Basically, if it's pickle-related, I want it in my mouth.

When I finally polish off a big, fat jar of Vlasic dill spears, I gaze down at the pint of mouthwatering pickle juice. And I want to drink the whole entire thing.

It's not like I've never enjoyed a mouthful of pickle juice. When I was drunk or hungover I especially liked to steal gulps from the jar in the refrigerator. I've weaned myself off my errant pickle juice desires, but now, pregnant, with a big salty green jar of it sitting on the counter, I am weak. But not too weak to grab my magic information screen, aka my smartphone, and quickly google "pregnant pickle juice."

And what do I find? Much like the sisterhood of compulsively masturbating pregnant women with vibrators, there also exists an online sisterhood of pregnant women who have complicated feelings about their desire to consume large quantities of pickle juice.

"I work in a deli," one stricken women writes, "and every day, when I transfer the pickles from the bucket to the jars, I drink about a quarter cup of the juice. Is this okay?!?!?!" I see myself in her shameful sipping and frantic cry for help. And her cry is answered! A chorus of vinegar-swilling pregnant women chime in about their own habits, encouraging her not to worry about it and drink that pickle juice with abandon!

"Maybe just drink a lot of water afterward," one prudent woman suggests, "to dilute the salt in your system, as the salt can be bloating."

I decide that's what I'll do. I fill up a mason jar with water. And then I pound the fuck out of that jar of pickle juice. It is, easily, the *best*-tasting, most cosmically satisfying thing I have ever ingested in my life. I feel like there is a halo of light radiating from the crown of my head, surrounded by sparkling, pickle-green stars. It was as if every desire one had ever had in one's life was satisfied at once. Forget the baby in my belly—right then, the reason I was pregnant was to make pickle juice taste *this good*.

I was pretty full after drinking the whole jar of Vlasic juice, but I did the right thing and sucked down the jar of water, hoping to undo any damage. Um, too little, too late. Already bloated from the onslaught of IVF hormones shot into my ass each night—not to mention the actual zygote swiftly growing in my uterus—the pickle juice pumps my bloatation up to a level I have never before experienced, like *that*. Orson soon comes home from work and finds me there in the kitchen, still sporting a residual high from the pickle juice, marveling at the size of my stomach.

"I drank pickle juice," I explained. "Look how bloated it made me!" I look about four months pregnant; I think I'm about four weeks. I wonder how I'm going to manage my new pickle juice habit and deal with the intense post-juice bloating, but as I have found to happen, this particular craving tapers off, and soon I'm not interested in pickles anymore.

OH NO. I HAVE THE ROTTENEST SINUS INFECTION EVER, AND IT'S BECAUSE I'M PREGNANT. Who knew about all the terrible things that befall pregnant people? I guess it's because the pregnant body produces so much mucus, and also everything—like, my entire body—is sort of swollen, so voilà, a sinus infection. I feel generally vulnerable to them, anyway, as a result of snorting all sorts of sketchy powders and liquids in my youth. I hope this isn't the start of nine months with an eyeball headache.

We have an appointment at the fertility clinic for an ultrasound peek. Sandra, the receptionist who is sort of obsessed with us and whom we are now similarly obsessed with, squeals with glee when she spots me and Orson. She peers at my face with her heavily eye-linered eyes.

"You're having a girl," she predicts.

"I am?"

"It's in your face," she says, and nods, fingering a medallion dangling around her neck. She flashes it at us. "Saint Benedict," she explains. "I'm Catholic."

Sandra might *think* she's Catholic, but like my mother and most of the other Catholic women in my family, what they all really are witches. Spooky ladies who know how to tell what sort of baby a person is having by the shape of their pregnant face. How to win the lotto by looking up what you dreamed last night in some ancient, numerical dream book, then playing the numbers ascribed to what you dreamed. Sandra is Mexican, and my family is a bunch of Euro mutts, but she might as well be my aunt or something.

As it happens, both my mother and my sister also think that I'm having a girl. I don't think much about anyone's guesses, but then my mother gives hers a perfectly spooky Catholic-witch twist. "I had a dream that I had a third grandchild," she says. "A girl. And they say you have the *opposite* of what you dream."

"So now you think I'm having a boy?" I ask her.

"I don't know . . ." Her voice trails off in an eerie singsong.

Who are "they," anyway?

At a support group for alcoholics that I attend, a woman I've never met holds my hand while we pray. I'm super attracted to this lady, in the particular way I am drawn to women of a certain age who look like they were crazy pill-popping sluts in their youth but are now sort of mellow and rich and have had some plastic surgery and wear interesting jewelry and keep their nails done and talk a little too loud. Possible narcissists, but something about them makes me want to be their audience, their little pet. This woman is so excited that I am pregnant, but when I tell her I am but two months pregnant, she screams like Yoko Ono and clasps her silk-scarf-draped chest.

"*Only* two months?" she cries, looking at my bulging belly.

"Yup," I say, and try to resist going into my spiel about how I did IVF and have been on and off fertility hormones for nine months and they really bloat you—none of it is any of her business and all of it makes me sound like I feel bad about looking so pregnant.

"You're going to have a big baby," the woman declares in this somber tone, as if she has predictive powers and is not just making the natural conclusion one would make at the sight of my belly. Because I am right and she is a narcissist, the focus doesn't stay on me for too long, and she goes on to talk all about how she had her daughters the Ayurvedic way.

Back to my belly. Slowly, through the past near year of hormone shots in my ass, I have been acquiring larger and larger pairs of $9.99 jeans from the Urban Outfitters sale rack, and have reached the point that I need a belly band, some sort of wide elastic loop that you pull up over the fly of your unzipped jeans so you can keep wearing them. Orson and I live near a mall that was recently called the "worst mall in America" on a Judgmental Map of San Francisco, and it has what is probably the worst Macy's in America, which is a bold claim, I know. Macy's seems like a great place to find one of these belly bands, so we set off toward our sad neighborhood mall.

I've been to this mall twice, once in the nineties, on a sad date with Tali, when we thought we could maybe date each other, wherein she bought me an Orange Julius, which I pretended to like because they seemed campy; and then again on New Year's Eve, when I was sick with my mysterious holiday illness and couldn't really go anywhere, to go to Macy's and then hit up the mall theater to watch *Blue Is the Warmest Color*.

Aside from me and Orson, the only people at the nine P.M. New Year's Eve screening of *Blue Is the Warmest Color* were another lesbian couple and a single man, who was probably masturbating. So my hopes aren't high for Macy's, and that is good, because it is pretty pathetic, with a minuscule maternity section in a cramped corner of the kids' floor. Amid the ugly clothes our woman-hating culture punishes pregnant people with, I do find a belly band, and I march it over to the cashier, talking Orson out of trying on pairs of children's Levi's along the way. (This is a known secret among people on the transmasculine spectrum: while clothing from the men's department is oftentimes too big, the larger clothing in the boys' section can fit like a charm.) I see the disappointment as Orson's shop-y desires get waved away, but I promise we can return when I'm a little further along and we both have cause to mill around the kid's section.

4.

TOTALLY JUSTIFIABLE
DAY SLEEPING

I love going to my appointments with Dr. Joan, my lesbian elder obstetrician. At least I *think* she's a lesbian. Being so gay in such a gay place for so long really does make everyone seem gay after a point. Dr. Joan asks about Orson, and our age difference comes up—nine years. "It's good to have a young person in your life," she says with a knowing little squint. Is Dr. Joan not only a lesbian elder obstetrician, but a lesbian elder obstetrician cougar?

I have to ask Dr. Joan if she will please, please, *please* give me an ultrasound so I can peek at the baby. She agrees, and we gasp and coo at the tiny being forming in my uterus. The heartbeat is strong and growth is on target.

Dr. Joan gives me an exam and makes the shocking pronouncement that I have a long, wide pelvis, excellent for childbirth. Never did I suspect such a thing about myself. I've been worried that childbirth will be difficult if not impossible—like, what if I'm just too small and the baby won't fit through the exit? All this time, my smallish body has been harboring a long, wide pelvis perfect for childbearing! It's wild how much hearing this changes my attitude about pushing a person out my nethers.

Dr. Joan asks if I have any questions, and I admit I am concerned about that one nipple I got pierced by a student at the cut-rate piercing studio, back in 1994, for twenty-five dollars. I haven't had a ring in it for decades, but I wonder if it will negatively impact my breastfeeding ability. Dr. Joan says nope; milk might come out *through* the piercing, but regardless, the baby will navigate around it. Then Dr. Joan drops some non-awesome news: I've gained too much weight too quickly, and I need to slow my (cinnamon) roll.

But I'm pregnant! Don't I get to just eat and eat and eat whatever I want? Dr. Joan shrugs. "You don't want to gain an extra ten pounds if you can help it," she says. But really—WHY NOT? I feel pretty good about just letting my hunger and my body do whatever, and just figuring it out (or not) after the baby is born.

"Just try to eat carrots, and hummus, and nuts," Dr. Joan suggests.

"Okay," I say, trying not to sulk. I deeply understand that food will never taste as good as it does right now, while pregnant. That does mean that carrots taste sweeter, hummus tastes creamier, and nuts taste like tangible reminders that the earth loves us. However. The thought of dropping my new pint-a-day ice cream habit fills me with hormonal rage.

I phone my mother on my way out of the building.

"I have to watch what I eat!" I cry. "I've gained too much too fast!" My mother commiserates with me, launching into her Tuna Fish Sandwich story, one she will continue to repeat throughout the duration of my pregnancy:

When my mother was pregnant with me, her doctor was super strict about only allowing her to gain some ridiculously small amount of weight, and when she came in to his office heavier than he wanted, he would scold her, because that was what doctors did to women in the early seventies. "I don't know how I gained so much," my mother said in her defense, to which the doctor replied, "I'll tell you how it happened—you put a knife in one hand and a fork in the other!"

"What an asshole!" I gasp at my mom, and she laughs. After that, she was sticking to a stricter diet, but after each weigh-in with Dr. Asshole, she would go to the deli and have a tuna fish sandwich, French fries, and a Coke. She lived for these afternoons, because tuna fish sandwiches, fries, and Cokes were all she wanted to eat while pregnant. My poor mom!

In the coming months, the Tuna Fish Story will be replaced by the Red Rocking Chair Story, when she repeatedly recounts how a "big Irish nurse" had allowed her to sit on the red leather rocking chair in her office while she was in labor. My mom stayed there, rocking and chain-smoking. Then she had to go back to her room, and her roommate was screaming in such pain that it gave my mom an anxiety attack. The big Irish nurse had gone home, and my mom, totally alone, finally asked for something for the pain.

"And give her something, too, please!" my mother begged about the screaming roommate, to which the nurse replied, "Oh, she's so high she doesn't even know where she is."

My mother got a shot in the butt and pushed me out a couple hours later. When the big Irish nurse came back to the hospital, she told my mom that if she'd only been able to stay by her side, my mother would have been able to do the whole labor med-free. But my mom didn't mind the meds: "They gave me a shot in the ass and I was flyin' high," she recounts happily. And there is the story of my birth.

ON THE WAY HOME FROM THE HOSPITAL, I STOP AT MY LOCAL CO-OP AND PICK up a bag of baby carrots and a thing of hummus. "Have you had this hummus before?" the man at the register enthuses. "It's amazing!"

I'm doubtful that any hummus can really be *that* amazing, and I really wish I was picking up a thing of cream cheese to be dipping my carrots in, but whatever. I do what the doctor tells me.

Being pregnant is totally exhausting, and I spend my entire second trimester doing something I *never* do: napping. Napping makes me feel like I stayed up all night on speed and my life is falling apart. It's a sign of depression, or being a resident of Portland, Oregon. Aside from visiting Portland and crashing from crystal meth, I don't nap, so this second trimester is a new landscape of totally justifiable day sleeping. Also, porn. My hormones are so out-of-control crazy, I *swear* I would sit down at my computer fully intending to write, then find myself on PornTube watching a video of a blindfolded woman tied to a giant block of ice, transfixed. I discover a whole subset of porn that fetishizes ballerinas, and then one where women pretend to be giant, floppy dolls.

And because I'm so exhausted, napping all the time, I find that I'm slowing down in other ways. Once I hit my third trimester, I'm canceling stuff once a week, asking people to fill in for me at events I've not missed in over a decade. I am very, very happy being pregnant: the crazy sensation of a little person swimming inside me, the free seats on the bus, the kindly way the world smiles at me. A totally new way to have a body—the giddy shock at seeing my belly get bigger . . . and bigger . . . and *bigger,* my mermaid tattoo stretched into a giant sea creature across my stomach. But although I am happy in my state, it is a state best enjoyed from the comfort of my living room while clutching a pint of Steve's Brooklyn Blackout ice cream, which I ate basically every day for a month straight. (Sorry, Dr. Joan.)

I think I'm ready to take on childbirth and push out this little person—a little dude, it turns out, per the existence of a teeny weenie spotted on the ultrasound, but I don't have to tell *you* how biological sex does not equal gender, so who knows how butch or femme this child will be. Orson and I begin shopping for a doula.

The first woman we interview comes highly recommended, but in our house she sits at our table, absentmindedly juggling our drink coasters, seeming super bored, saying things like, ". . . Yeah, I guess I can take you on." I don't like feeling as if I am putting out a person I will be paying, like, *a thousand dollars* to help me through one of the most important moments of my life, so we pass.

The next doula we interview is actually a doula *duo,* a pair of the blondest, most traditionally beautiful young doula women ever to coax a baby from a womb. Together, they are a spectacle. I couldn't tell how this would work for me in childbirth. Maybe their beauty would be a balm, like a walking bouquet of flowers, something to meditate upon? They try to sell their partnership as a two-for-the-price-of-one bargain, explaining that most doulas get so exhausted during a long labor, the quality of service dips when you need it most. They would relieve each other when they got sleepy, promising a fresh, doe-eyed doula at all times. This made sense, but I couldn't help thinking that they were weaklings. Give me a tough-ass doula with stamina to match my own, both of us delirious and sweaty and crazed with birth. Who wants a pretty little pony doula trotting into your birthing room all showered and rested, when you have crossed over into some sort of endurance zone known only to prisoners of war and people squeezing out babies?

The doula we end up choosing is like a cross between the intense PFLAG mother from *Queer as Folk* and a woman reading auras at a psychic fair. In other words, she is *perfect.* A Libra with a halo of cherry-cola curls, she is probably in her sixties, wears groovy sunglasses, has some Celtic tattoos, and is a shaman. As part of prepping me for labor, I visit her office for a vision quest. I sit on a puffy recliner, blindfolded, and am hypnotized until the spirit of Great Motherhood is revealed to me in the form of a turtle. It makes sense that the Great Mother would appear to me as a turtle, for I have spent many summers on the Yucatán watching sea turtles lug themselves onto the shore, laboriously digging a nest with their unwieldy turtle flippers, laying a bunch of Ping-Pong turtle eggs, then lumbering back into the sea.

As I continued to meet with my doula, working out a birth plan with her guidance, a simple fact becomes harder to ignore. My baby is breech. The clock ticks, days pass, he stays this way. There are many things you can do to try to encourage a *bébé* to get into position. I do sloppy, improper inversions against my couch. I speak to the baby, begging him to flip. I locate the most abrasive Hole song I can source, the excellent "Teenage Whore," and lay it upon my belly, trying to irritate him toward my crotch. I weaponize a bag of frozen peas, placing them on his head to drive him toward a warmer climate. I get acupuncture and am prescribed the Chinese medicine moxibustion. I even agree to an ECV—external cephalic version, also called, simply, version.

ECV is a procedure wherein you are given a shot to relax your uterus, and then three grown adults put their full weight on your pregnant stomach, lifting the baby up inside you and attempting to twist it around with their hands. If this sounds hideous and terrifying, it's because it is. It is also my last shot at having a "natural"— i.e., vaginal—birth, and with all the pressure on the modern pregnant person to forgo the Labor Industrial Complex, wherein one is plied with drugs that numb you from the waist down, or artificially instigate your labor, sometimes with the help of a *vacuum* that attempts to dislodge the stubborn *bébé* from the womb.

The Labor Industrial Complex, we've now long been told, cares about efficiency and doctors' schedules, and has cut itself off from the natural rhythm of each individual birth. Ever since medicine kicked midwives out of the picture, midwives and other more natural-oriented birth workers, such as doulas, have been fighting their way back in, advocating for a return to labor that is, yes, more painful, but also more in synch with what is ultimately best for the baby and the parent, pushing for mindfulness, presence, and time-honored techniques over a doped-up labor rife with unnecessary interventions.

I knew moms both online and IRL who equate C-section with a sort of failure, who risk their lives with home births gone askew, or submit to the surgery but flagellate themselves for it later—much like the moms who have a hard time breastfeeding, another facet of parenting to which moral judgment has been assigned, in spite of its success or failure hinging on biological factors mostly out of your own control.

But as much as I am hoping for a natural birth, the reality starts to settle in: I have a nine-pound baby in my uterus, seemingly sitting in lotus position, comfy as hell and not willing to budge. And sure, I have a doula, a "mindful childbirth class," a medical team, and a mom culture insisting on exhausting all efforts for a vaginal birth. But I also have a hairdresser, a classy and stylish modern femme, who exhorts the luxury of the C-section, who deems the drugs prescribed totally excellent, the healing bedrest dreamy, and her unscathed vagina priceless. As I had been influenced by her style and fashion choices, so I cannot help but be a little swayed by this portrait of a C-section as a type of spa treatment.

But to the ECV I go. My doula comes along, and I am deeply grateful for her presence—maternal but with a misfit, outcast vibe I groove on. I feel as though she casts a protective energy around me, that if anything were to go awry, she will know it before the doctors do. As I lie upon a medical table, she stands at my head, rubbing my temples and encouraging me to breathe.

I should mention that having my temples rubbed, my head pet, my hair played with—it's all my favorite things on earth. Maybe even better than sex, which I do heartily enjoy. I think it is maybe worth it to go through this grotesque procedure just to have my temples so expertly rubbed by a shaman.

The mindfulness techniques, which I may or may not get to

put into practice during labor, sure do come in handy while three full-grown humans dig their hands deep into my abdomen, connecting with my lazy-ass child and pulling, scooping, twisting, shoving him around in the giant sac of my belly. *Breathe, breathe,* soothed my doula. Aside from one horrifying glance, I keep my eyes squished closed, count my breaths like I'd learned to at the Zen Center, the way I'd done during the more painful parts of all my tattoos. Orson clutches my hand supportively, but I have seen the distressed look in their eyes, and know how ill-equipped they are, constitutionally, to deal with the horrors of having a body, and feel sure that after seeing my once-cute tummy now shockingly engorged with life and being yanked and swung around by a team of doctors—well, our romantic life, sadly, will never be the same.

The doctors all agree that no one has ever sailed through this medieval procedure with the calm grace I displayed, counting and breathing beneath the soothing ministrations of my doula. My inner child, chronically hungry for praise from authority figures, radiates with glee. The swell of cheer at my meditative prowess soon abates, replaced by the somber confirmation that the ECV has not worked, my baby refuses to get off his ass, and although some hardcore adrenaline junkies *do* attempt to vaginally deliver a breech baby, the size of this kid plus the narrowness of my pelvis ensure that I'd die an eighteenth-century-style death if I attempted it. I feign disappointment until out of reach of the doctors, and then clutch Orson with relief. I don't break out a bottle of champagne—I'm sober! And pregnant!—but I do go for a celebratory scoop of ice cream. I am having a C-section after all.

5.

A TENDER ALIEN

At Shaman Doula's urging, I decide to wait to go into labor naturally, resisting the annoyed medical personnel, skeptical and confused as to why I am putting such a premium on this barbaric experience. My doula insists that allowing your body to go into labor before a C-section is good for my hormones, as well as for the baby's lungs. Having been at the mercy of my hormones since puberty, I want to do right by them as much as possible. And, bizarrely, I want the experience of water breaking between my legs, tsunami-ing out from me all over a sidewalk, like Charlotte in the *Sex and the City* movie.

But my baby seems pretty happy right where he is. Too content to instigate labor.

In the days leading up to my due date, and the days trailing away from it, I obsessively track the twinges and cramps that shoot through my abdomen. I make frequent treks to the hospital, where I lie with various monitors stuck to my body, tracking heartbeat and contractions, only to be sent home—but not without an offer to get a C-section on the books. I exist in a strange limbo, excited for a future that seems poised to burst at any moment, nostalgic for the rarefied state—pregnancy—that is slipping away. I visualize my mer-baby, swimming side to side in my enormous belly. Sometimes I feel a kick on my right side, and I give him a friendly poke, only to feel him *swish* over to the left, and kick me again. I respond with a poke. We go on like this for a bit, and I realize that we are playing, my baby and me. Playing our first game together. What a fairy tale, to have a creature alive inside of you! I am a benevolent monster, a tender alien, the most primally human I'd ever be. I want it to last forever.

EVENTUALLY, IT ISN'T MY CRAMPS BRINGING ME INTO THE HOSPITAL, IT IS THE doctors, insisting on checking on me each day. To be beyond your due date, the baby continuing to grow inside you, shifts you into ever riskier territory. I have a Sagittarius stellium in the fifth house that prevents me from ever really believing anything bad will happen to me, in spite of however many bad things *have* ever happened to me, so I feel fancy-free each time I waddle in to have my cervix prodded, but I am beginning to feel guilty for putting out the medical workers, who grow warier and warier as I breeze in and out without officially getting a C-section on the books. To them it is a question between a chill, preplanned surgery or an urgent one performed in the midst of a crisis. Am I putting my baby in physical danger, letting him hang out in my uterus for so long? I certainly am putting him in astrological danger.

The days are passing, we are moving deeper into fall, Halloween decorations are now scattered about the landscape. And each day, the sun shimmies a little deeper into the outskirts of Libra, sidling up to Scorpio. And it isn't just the sun. The moon, Venus, and Mars *all* have invites to the Scorpio party happening on October twenty-third, just *two days* away, from where I lie on a cot. Once more, the medical folks try to intervene on what to them appears to be a privileged modern woman hell-bent on experiencing a nineteenth-century childbirth.

"Do you think you're ready to meet your baby today?" a nurse sweetly inquires. "We've got the time for it. What do you think?"

I am in no hurry to "meet" my baby, enjoying as I am this strange bonding I am doing with him as he nests inside my body. But I get full-body shivers at the thought of giving birth to a baby with a Scorpio stellium. A Scorpio Sun, cool, fine. But *four planets* in that gothic sign? There would even be an *eclipse,* a sort of Scorpionic Battle Royale between the sun and the moon, and no, I did not want to die upon the operating table.

After agreeing to have my baby that very day, after summoning a flummoxed Shaman Doula, who is perhaps irritated that I have succumbed to the Labor Industrial Complex, I sit in a small room, my bum hanging out of my threadbare hospital gown, and call my beloved sister, Madeline.

"Is it so terrible that I am doing this?" I demand of her. The truth is, I *loved* Scorpios. Yes, they're paranoid, prone to nervous disorders, nurturing of grudges, know-it-all mansplainers regardless of their genders. But in so many ways, Scorpios seem to be engaging with life on this existential plane with more chutzpah and sincerity than any other sign. Why would I deliberately take this astrological birthright away from my son, instead condemning him to the shallow, codependent, neurotic life of a Libra?

"You're doing the right thing," my sister, traitor to her sign, assures me. "Just having your sun in Scorpio can be a lot. And you're talking about four planets."

"And an eclipse," I remind her.

"And he'll have testosterone in his body," she reminds me.

"Ugh," I shudder, remembering a musician I once toured with, a cisgender guy with a Scorpio stellium who was a sex addict with a rigorous (and public) masturbation regimen.

I rack my brain for other Scorpio stelliums I have known. There was my coworker at a Marin County brothel, a heavily augmented woman who deeply loved both her hooker job and her boyfriend, a marine who hadn't the foggiest as to how she paid the bills. It seemed like tempting fate to catch you in a compromising situation was a hallmark of a Scorpio stellium, no?

But then I recall my dear, old friend Frank, a transwoman who makes her living reading tarot cards and communing with books, a performance artist who channels the resentful ghosts of overrated Beat poets, whose youthful occupation at a lip-synch-y drag bar earned her a reputation more fearsome than that of Courtney Love, as she was known to knock glasses off tables, knock tables onto patrons, and give lap dances that resulted in a trip to the emergency room. Sigh. Frank had both a Scorpio stellium *and* testosterone in her body, and I could not imagine an individual I'd be prouder to parent. But. Still. Maybe I'll get a radical genderqueer witch, or maybe I'll get a flasher in a raincoat. And anyway, the notion of a surgery during an eclipse has me more spooked than a Puritan lost in the woods of Salem. I embrace my decision. I embrace my little baby Libra, a peacemaker, able to see both sides, drawn to art and music and romance, beholden to beauty. An air sign, like me, we will gab and gab, I will take him to thrift stores and let him pick out vintage caftans for me. Sure, maybe Libras are codependent, but I could make that work for me. I was gunning for a mama's boy, after all. I thank my sister for her wisdom and wait to be swept away to the operating room.

It doesn't happen.

The calm day at the hospital has taken a sudden turn into chaos. Emergency C-sections, the fate the staff had been urging me away from all these days, have erupted all around me. The nurse asks me to go home and return the following day.

"It will be better anyway," she tries to persuade me, after having finally succeeded at persuading me to stay. "You'll be rested, and you can fast and come in first thing in the morning."

One more night to experience my baby living on the inside of me. One more night of hazy, sleepless sleep in my unwieldy body, sweating naked, clamped around my enormous curling pregnancy pillow, jolted out of dreams by the force of my snores, my right hand with its weirdly triggered carpal tunnel pain wrapped in a Velcro mitt. Sure, why not. The planets will still be in Libra come morning.

6.

HI, BABY

The *Groundhog Day*–esque nature of my recent days—a gentle cramping in my uterus, the trek to the hospital, the gloved finger insulting my cervix, the same-old sonogram—hits a déjà vu peak the following morning, as I lie on a bed, in my buttless johnnie, an IV port jammed into the crook of my arm, listening as a nurse explains that the delivery rooms are again packed with emergency C-sections and could I please go back home and try again tomorrow?

The irony, if that's what it is, of dodging the delivery room for weeks, the staff practically begging to slice the baby out of me, only to finally capitulate and then be sent home and then sent home again—well, it didn't exactly register on me, bleary as I was from a night of no sleep and a morning of no coffee. The astrological clock was ticking. Was it his destiny, this child, to be born on the first day of Scorpio, during a planetary avalanche of intense sex-and-death energy? The nurse finally agrees that if I was fine with waiting in that hospital room for, *oh*, like eight more hours, they could probably get to me around dinnertime. I curl up on the starchy, white hospital bedding and, trying not to bump the IV port sticking grotesquely from my arm, wrap my arms around my belly and take a nap.

At dinnertime, I am brought into the operating room, alone, for my spinal. It is jabbed into my body by a student even though I had pleaded in my birth plan to please please *please* not have students doing things like sticking needles into my spine. But whatever—it's not a birth *plan,* it's a birth *intention.* Morphine starts flowing into my IV port, which I notice by becoming, suddenly, really fucking high. It feels amazing. Then there is Orson, in scrubs, leaning their head down by my head, kissing me and speaking in hushed, excited tones. *Are you okay how are you feeling are you ready oh my god can you believe it?*

I knew that there would be a sheet of sorts draped across me, protecting me from the grisly sight of my insides being cut open—something one should never have to see—but I always imagined it as a delicate little block of white, like an elegant clothesline hung above my waistline. In fact, it is more like a giant blue tarp, and it is about an inch from my face. My body is tilted at an incline, and my arms are stretched out like Christ on the cross (they had honored my birth *intention* of not strapping them down). The doctor made little cuts into my skin and asked if I could feel them, and not only could I not feel them, I didn't even fucking care, because morphine is so wonderful.

Orson feels both very close and very far, an effect of the drug. I am pondering this when the sudden cry of an actual baby fills the room. "Oh my god," I say. "Go to him, go to the baby, go."

They kiss me and are gone. I float in a woozy state of awe, knowing there is a baby here now, that it has been inside me and is mine. The faraway feeling keeps growing, like time and space are stretching out in front of me. Oh my god, there is my baby's face. His lips are so red, they are rubies, they are fairy tale lips.

"Say something to him," Orson says, holding the squinting newborn over me. What does one say to a baby? "Hi, baby," I say. "Hi, Atticus." Orson and the baby are whisked away to the nursery, and Shaman Doula is brought in to be by my side. She goes into a slight trance to communicate with the baby, and relays to me that his guardian animal spirit is a turtle, and that he loves water and would always want to be near water, to feel the current. Then she tells me she's seen a dragonfly. She is still being witchy—there are no insects in the operating room. Still, this is interesting.

"That's my grandfather," I say.

My mother believes that her father shows his spirit to her in the form of dragonflies, which she spots constantly, hovering with their iridescent helicopter wings. The doula squeezes my shoulders. I am impressed with her psychic acumen. Her vision lent credence to my mother's faith, and now I believe my grandfather is present in the operating room in the form of an invisible dragonfly. I hope that he did not arrive from the land of the dead to take me back with him; that stretchy space-time feeling has not stopped. I continue to feel like I am being pulled farther away from where I am.

I announce to whoever is listening that I am about to throw up. A little blue sock of sorts, with accordion folds, is held under my mouth to catch the upchuck. I can barely twist my head to reach it, and puke down my face. Who cares, I feel great, I had a baby. There is an intellectual sensation, a thought, I guess, that maybe I should be worried, what with the elasticity of space-time and the vomiting and all. But I can't muster up the corresponding emotion of worry, not while surrounded with a team of medical professionals who are actually being paid cash money to worry about me while I bliss out on the best freelapse of my life.

"She isn't looking good," the shaman doula alerts my team.

"She's losing blood," I hear someone say. No big deal. I mean, I'm in an operating room, surrounded by surgeons. If I am going to lose a lot of blood, this is the place to do it.

I am soon rolled into my recovery room, the ceiling lights passing above my head in a glowing highway of sorts. It seems the problem with my body has been sorted, but alarm at my lost blood rises again. Another flock of people—doctors, nurses, students—gather around me, fussing. An ultrasound machine is rolled in, to see if any tissue was accidentally left inside me, I'm informed. It is cute that people are still speaking to me as if I am a whole and cognizant person and not just a gossamer thread blowing in the breeze, *in the world but not of it*, like a Jehovah's Witness.

I manage to ask my doula for my glasses, and she sets the frames gently on my nose. I can't feel the ultrasound wand sliding over my belly, what with the recent spinal injection; the glowing green pixels on the screen mean nothing. A doctor tells me my womb is clean, but if I don't stop bleeding, they are going to have to give me a transfusion. Was I okay with that? *Totally.* Did transfusions come with additional morphine? I wondered. Someone gives me a shot to stop the bleeding, and I notice I am wearing these giant anti-blood-clot boots on my legs and they are giving my calves what look like a fabulous massage. Can I stay here forever?

Even though I know I am possibly dying, I feel very great and can't take *seriously* the thought that I might die, what with my opiate-enhanced optimism. Orson walks into the room, our brand-new baby all bundled in their arms. They look at me, at the urgent rush of doctors, and their face grows tight with alarm. A nurse grabs their arm and gently herds them out of the way. Somehow I roll my head to face them, lift my arm, and give them a big thumbs-up and a toothy smile. I need them to know that I know I am going to be fine, even though I also know I could maybe die. They don't really respond to my thumbs-up, as they are too distracted by the sudden realization that I could maybe die, so I do it again, and then maybe again, until they acknowledge it with a small, scared smile. And, obviously, I am right and I totally don't die.

Once the medical team approves my morphine-induced optimism and confirms that I am okay, the bleeding has stopped, the urgent hubbub around me falls quiet, and my doula rushes in with an urgency of her own.

"Put the baby on her, put the baby on her," she directs, clearly feeling that too much time has already elapsed between the baby's emergence into the world and the orienting skin-to-skin contact so many believe to be crucial for mother-baby bonding. The baby's hot little body, undone from his bunting, is placed on my own sweaty chest, and I marvel at the animal I have become, have always been, as he moves instinctively to my nipple and begins to nurse. My body makes *food!* I love when the most natural things are also the most magical, the most incredible. Colostrum, the thick, nutrient-dense pre-milk, nicknamed liquid gold for its buttermilk hue and superfood powers, leaches from my areola, like I am some kind of primordial mother-goddess.

There is yet another idea behind this deep, animal contact I am enjoying with my baby, and that is epigenetics. I am fascinated by the newish science, the idea that trauma can be passed down through family lines and, therefore, can also be healed, cycles broken, through closeness and care. I think about the lineage of mental illness that has traveled down my matrilineal line, going back at least to my great-grandmother, who married an abusive husband; how she transferred that trauma onto my grandmother, who was forced to dash to the police station to save her mother's life; how she was plagued with nightmares of her father and suffered a nervous breakdown when my own mother was only five; the trauma of that for my mom added to the fact that my grandmother was a rather cruel parent, being freaked out all the time as she was, no coping skills and what not. And how later, my mother was coached by the science of the time not to breastfeed us, me and my sister, my poor sister starved for early maternal contact for days after her birth, as my mother had come down with a cold, and the hospital feared her sickening her offspring. It is also so much to consider, the early effects of parental bonding. If you think about it, and I did think about it, mightily, during those profound early days of motherhood, most everyone gets off to a rather traumatic start, birth itself being a trauma, perhaps, and then everything that may or may not follow it: the home you are taken back to, mine thick with cigarette smoke and my angsty, alcoholic dad, so wounded that *his* dad was petty and resentful enough to refuse to come and see me, his granddaughter, that my father took a knife and stabbed it through a box of pasta that had been sitting on the table, triggering my grandmother, who was there, filling the house with cigarette smoke as they all were, and how my grandmother had to leave then, disturbed by my father's drama with the knife, and who can blame her. And there I am in the midst of it, a tiny baby, soaking in the vibes, various genes being turned on or lying dormant according to the care I need and if I receive it or not. And I did get my ancestral anxiety, not to mention my father's alcoholism, and I imagine myself as a tiny switchboard being lit up by these hapless grown-ups, who'd been at the mercy of their own errant switchboards for far too long.

I hadn't consciously had my baby as a way to release ancestral trauma. But in my postpartum state, which, even without the pain-killers is a deeply psychedelic one, it seems that birthing a baby and working with it to heal epigenetic trauma, placing a consciously birthed and nurtured human onto the planet, can possibly be a radically helpful act.

And so I move to soothe my baby's every cry, am moved to him with surges of hormones, new feelings inside my body that remain there even today, at the sound of his tears or distress. I have to—it seems imperative, essential. I find it hard to explain to those who haven't experienced childbirth; it can seem like a parenting philosophy you're adhering to, or a motherly impulse to smother, over-parent. But I can't stress enough the power of new chemicals that the baby has unleashed inside my body, and how totally physical the need to tend to him is, to feed him when hungry, soothe him when screaming, bring us back to our joined equilibrium, mother and baby soothing each other, and maybe, possibly, an epigenetic legacy of hurt being thinned to vanishing. With my baby peacefully upon my body, I learn a new feeling: like euphoria, but calmer, or like contentment, but mind-blowing. Language fails, but that makes a sort of sense. This experience is prelanguage, ancient and primal.

7.

SOMETHING HAS FLIPPED

For three nights, as I remained hospitalized and healing, the baby slept in Orson's arms, as Orson slept in a makeshift bed cobbled together from a couple chairs. Atticus stared at his baba with an intensity that seemed far too alert for someone so recently born. He remained that way—focused, intense, alert. A good baby, one who doesn't really fuss too much, though we were trying not to label the basic having of emotions as good or bad. He does scream like we're murdering him when we change his diaper. It makes me think of his stubborn seat inside me, his refusal to invert no matter the techniques we applied. This lounging, Venus-ruled Libra won't ever like being told to move.

Everything has changed since I came home from the hospital. The house looks like the furniture was rearranged in our absence, but then put back where it had been, a sort of uncanny, underground hum, a backbeat of deep transfiguration. I remember how space-time seemed to shift with the onset of drugs, and how it intensified as too much blood left my body. Perhaps I had crossed over dimensions, into another version of my life. It was trippy enough to make sense. How in the world did I—messy and poor, addict and queer, slutty, weird, unstable—wind up here, in this veritable cottage, one with a white picket fence, with a baby in my arms? The very air around me felt changed.

The days after Atticus's arrival had an ease, a sleep-deprived, delirious ease. I'm relieved of my constant need to brainstorm for work, to come up with a clever fund-raising idea or an innovative new creative project. I don't have to curate a performance or sell a bunch of magazine editors on my pitches. When the baby cries, I feed him, or I change his diaper, or I bounce him on the big orange fitness ball, or I walk back and forth, swinging and humming and shushing. When the baby doesn't cry, I put him on a blanket and wag a toy in his face. I put him on his belly and watch his neck get strong as it struggles to lift his head. I read him *The Snowy Day* and *Princess Smartypants* and *Big Red Barn* and also *Happy Punks 1 2 3* and *A is for Activist*.

Those weeks after birth, I thought my love—a brand-new, searing, scorching, unbearable love, not only for him, but for Orson—I thought this love would kill me. Why had no one told me about this love? How would I bear it? It was so beautiful that it was a pain inside me.

And we're all going to die, I couldn't help thinking, again and again. It was the hormones, the terrible vanishing of them, an elevator with a cut cord dropping not just to where I was prepregnancy, pre-ART hormone injections and patches, but down below my natural base level, whatever that was. I was plunged deep into some primordial prehormonal ooze I had never been in before. *We're all going to die someday,* I thought, a notion that tugged a whole new emotion in its wake. *The three of us will die. How can that be when we are here right now, so powerfully bound by this powerful love?*

The hormones would right themselves, more or less, over time, but still my eyes will well up when this thought intrudes. I never knew for certain that death was real before, had privately thought that I might live forever. I know how absurd this sounds, but I felt it inside me as a kind of truth nonetheless. Now something has flipped. There is a love as big as planets circling my heart, but the trade-off is a new comprehension that someday we all will be gone.

2021

AFTERWORD

All's well / Ends well

You would think that such an otherworldly reckoning with loss would have made it simpler, less devastating, when Orson left our marriage six years later, but alas, I did sob in the shower and sob snottily onto the cigarettes I smoked alone, late at night on the front steps. These moments echoed back to that overwhelming, prescient love I'd felt those first few weeks as a family. Had I felt our end there, in the liminal space of our beginning? Childbirth is so strange; again, I remember Exene saying it had made her more psychic. While my child experienced his birth, I had been somewhat close to death, and what was either phenomena, really? Where had my baby come from, and where would I have gone? In the midst of this remarkable moment, perhaps I could feel our dissolution begin. Surely, Orson and I had been brought together to bring this child into the world. Now that our work was finished, the undoing slowly began.

I think I'm mostly repaired from it all, although writing such a book in the shadow of a divorce is certainly a bizarre experience.

The impulse to keep intact the heart-eyes I had at the time butted up against something raw and hurt—and resentful. I wanted to bring you a beautiful queer love story. Does learning that something so seemingly unique and precious died the same quotidian death most relationships do—gone stale like a pastry one forgets to put in the fridge, vulnerable to rot and mold and betrayal and lies—ruin the tale? Does the sight of it broken in the garbage erase the memory of how delicious it was at its most fresh?

Perhaps the biggest hurdle, in the wake of a marriage you'd convinced yourself was the stuff of true fairy tales, is to allow yourself to suspend disbelief *again*. But, readers, I have. Typing this from the now, I can overhear my new partner, TJ, one room away planning our engagement party. Yes, I'd broken up with him countless times, so disturbed was I by his unbroken heart, his ability to simply love me and believe that the love meant something—was noble, strong enough to build a life on. *How naive,* I would sometimes think; then, *How heroic. What a paragon. What a dauntless model for having a heart.* I came to my senses and moved him into mine. One of my favorites of his many tattoos is a humble stick and poke high up on his legs reading *All's well / Ends well.* And I believe that.

My baby is now a little boy, seven going on eight, soon to start second grade. Currently he is spending the week at his other house, and this is a relief, as we have just returned—my boy, my fiancé, and myself—from a hectic trip up the East Coast, eating Italian ice and swimming in the Atlantic. While I initially despaired at losing half of my time with my child to a fifty–fifty custody arrangement, I have learned how totally *not* disagreeable it is to be a part-time parent. I get time alone to delve deep into work, steal cigarettes on the front porch, have epic sex and naked cuddles with my fiancé. I get to see friends: I live in Los Angeles now, and for a moment both Rhonda and Harris lived here as well, and though that makeshift, tender bond between the three of us never completely reformed, neither did it dissipate. Always, the echo of our embarking on a rarefied and queer experience—one that required a level of trust that we all instinctively *knew* we could have in one another—always, will that be there, triggering deep affection. I see Rhonda often enough, usually stark naked at a Korean spa or clinking seltzer bottles at parties; I see Quentin less, now that he has relocated to a professorship in the desert, his long years of study behind him as he transfers his knowledge to young people *so lucky* to have this particular queer intelligence at their disposal. All the while he remains Miss Super Extra Deluxe Pandemonium, who is not only an integral part of the drag queen story hours that have sprung up in libraries around the globe but also an author of the sorts of queer children's books read at such events. The last time I saw Quentin was on a visit to his desert environs, when he got to meet TJ, and the three of us ate fake-meat sandwiches and drank cactus sodas and bobbed in a hotel swimming pool after dark. Sometimes, when he smiles, his face becomes that of my child's and my heart can hardly stand the bolt of joy.

When my kid returns to me, our time takes on a sharper quality than before the divorce; it demands connection, intentionality. The hugs I insist upon when he leaves are more justifiable when I know I won't see him for days, though still he squirms away from me with shrieks when I grab him, and demands that I let him *lick my arm* (!) each time I insult him with a kiss.

"That's not the same!" I argue. "Licking is gross!"

"Well, I think kisses are gross," he states calmly, arms folded. Touché.

The weeks he lives with me inside the home we—Mama and TJ, Nana and the doggie, the two cats, the hamster living large in a three-story rodent cage—all share, we slide easily into our habits. Watching YouTube, with its parade of bros taping each other to the walls of their YouTuber mansions, racing RC cars, exploding multicolor rainbows of elephant toothpaste—this is for mornings only, when I sit beside my son on the couch, a coffee in hand, a stack of books beside me on the cushions. He loves these dudes, and I have learned to tolerate them. He is quick to share science facts and trivia with me, responding to my genuine awe at his knowledge bank with "I learned it on YouTube!" and a smile, his two front teeth taking their sweet time growing in. His hair a shaggy mullet, choppy bangs around his shining eyes, this little face I love so much it hurts. I'm not going to take his YouTube away.

Or his candy. It lives in the bottom of a kitchen cabinet, a realm referred to as "the candy stash." I use astrology to console myself when I feel alarm at his blatant hoarding of sweets. He's a Libra, child of Venus, goddess of sugar and all things delectable. Having a collection is a joy, is it not? I have only to look at my own shelves of books (so many unread!), my trays of crystals. He has bins of gummies, his favorite, in every formation: chicken's feet, watermelon slices, sharks, bottles of cola, fish, cherries. A bin for lollipops, his favorite being Tootsie Pops, though he is also partial to those giant multicolor swirls. They look like joke lollipops, they are so huge, and I mostly never let him eat them, to which he whines, "Then why did you get it for me?" and to which I reply, "I don't know," though I do, I do, of course I know, and it is because I cannot resist the urge to delight him any more than he can resist his urge to collect sugar.

He always asks me before he eats his candy, which I find darling, really, since he could easily be sneaking sweets from his stash left and right, but he does not. He is such a good boy, wicked as all seven-year-olds are: he loves to prank and has a special "prank bag" in his closet stuffed with eavesdropping tools and spy sunglasses and rubbery mounds of fake poop and cockroaches. He's naughty in that way, but also such a strident follower of rules, and what mother would not love such a thing, especially a mother not so prone to following the rules herself?

Weekday mornings, when he awakens at my house, our walk to school always includes the doggie and takes us by houses and grass and trees and cactus. He always stops to marvel at the one stretch where there are so many ants and to treat me to some YouTube ant trivia. I love this morning stroll, and I love the afternoon pickup stroll, too, even though it is much hotter by then, and the doggie will plop onto the ground in protest, and we will feed her water and watch the children from his school pass by us, some of them turning to say hello to my child, to say his name, and my child says *hi* back, and oh my gosh, he's making *friends,* a strange mixture of excitement and relief lights up my chest, and I rub his head or flip the long tail of his hair through my fingers, which he protests, immediately grumpy, and tells me that when he is taller than me he is going to do the same to me, see how I like it, and, honestly, I can't wait.

At home, he makes art, corralling whatever adult is free to join him at the little art table TJ has set up for him. Mostly he draws dragons, bulky and fierce, their wings curling, their toothed jaws spitting weapons native to their element: fireballs from the fire dragons, water from the water dragons, fruiting apple trees from the earth dragons, thick balls of dust from the dust dragons. He tries to sell them to us for exorbitant amounts of money, and sometimes succeeds. He loves math and boxing. He loves to ride the ocean on his belly, and he loves to wrestle. Sometimes he holds his hands like little paws, bent at the wrists; sometimes he meows rather than talks. He has a family of stuffed sloths who live on a shelf in his room. He plays shooter video games I swore I'd never allow; he's shockingly good at them. A world of Magna-Tiles, populated by all sorts of figurines and deemed Cutieland, lives on a foldout table in a storage room. Every night we read books, whatever gross series marketed to middle school boys we happen to be in the midst of, plus something nonfiction about animals. I like to do voices. He is still young enough to want company in the bathroom when he's sitting on the toilet. I perch on a stool on the other side of the room, and we play a game called Underball, where we throw his underwear back and forth, slingshotting the waistband or packing it into a fluffy orb and chucking it. He dares me to aim for his face, and I do have great aim. Downstairs, TJ and my mother can hear our loud guffaws. The other night I told him that I knew he would not want me in the bathroom with him forever, and that I was going to miss Underball when the time came. An expression I'd never seen flashed across his face, and he nodded and said, "I will, too."

I had a child so that I could experience the most that this earthly plane offers up for us. I wanted to feel the most of my body. I wanted to experience new levels of love. I got all of that, and more than I bargained for. The outer reaches of love, where it hits the limits of our understanding, where it merges into the Universe; a love whose seeming ability to transcend time reminds us that we do not even know what time is. I would live a million lives to be this child's mother again and again. I would roam as a ghost and protect his earthly body until he joined me—I mean, I will, Goddess willing, that's exactly what I'll do. My body is now changed forever, and so is my psyche, my capacity for love, my connection to the cosmos and to the depth of my ignorance as to what it all means. What is this experience, this earthly plane, these bodies? Motherhood is psychedelic.

At night, I lie with him until he falls asleep, and he singsongs my name softly—*Mama, Mama, Mama*—he asks me to cuddle him tightly, to scratch his back with my fingernails. He insists that he loves me more than I could ever love him, that he loves me *infinity*, and since he said it first, I just have to accept it and be so massively loved. I have learned not to argue, and so I nestle into him, all of my limbs wrapping around him, carrying him into sleep, both of us drifting off on a current of infinite love. Eventually, he won't need me to lie with him at night; he's already reading me the bedtime stories I've long read him. Eventually, he won't cry out in the night for me, won't climb into my lap when he burns his finger on a fresh-from-the-toaster Pop-Tart. The loss of these sweet moments, I have to believe, will be replaced by new ones: a stronger ability to have deep conversations, the joy of watching his real-life accomplishments, the continuous unfurling of this one human's personality, with all its strengths and challenges, its quirky interests, little peeks into the workings of his brain as it develops, as he becomes more and more the person he is meant to be. I get a front-row seat to all of it. To the astounding and mundane mystery of life, encapsulated in one little boy. What could be luckier.

ACKNOWLEDGMENTS

Thanks to Emily McCombs for being an early supporter of this concept. So much wild appreciation to Alison Lewis for taking me on with such enthusiasm. Thanks to my fantastic team at Dey Street—Carrie Thornton, Peter Kispert, Rosy Tahan, Heidi Richter, and Kate Napolitano—who the universe brought back into my life for another book! Special thanks for Vera Blossom for her help on the manuscript. Thanks to my sister and best friend, Kathleen Black, without whom this book would not exist. To Harris Kornstein, certainly the most generous person in the world, and to Tara Jepsen, one of the bravest. To Dashiell Lippman for the collaboration. To the moms and parents who supported my desire to have a baby when it still seemed like a possibly insane choice—Camille Roy, Jennifer Fink, Aya de Leon, Joey Soloway, Maggie Nelson, my former AA sponsor (you know who you are), and my own mother, Theresa Tomasik. To the friends who probably never stopped thinking it was an insane choice, but supported me anyway—Ali Liebegott, Beth Pickens, Tamara Llosa-Sandor, Clement Goldberg, Nicole J. Georges, and Deez Nutsian.

Thanks to TJ Payne for staying near and being true; my dark prince forevermore.

ABOUT THE AUTHOR

Michelle Tea is the author of more than a dozen books, including the cult-classic *Valencia*, the essay collection *Against Memoir*, and the speculative memoir *Black Wave*. She is the recipient of awards from the Guggenheim, Lambda Literary, and Rona Jaffe foundations; PEN/America; and other institutions. *Knocking Myself Up* is her latest memoir.

Tea's cultural interventions include brainstorming the international phenomenon Drag Queen Story Hour, cocreating the Sister Spit queer literary performance tours, and occupying the role of founding director at RADAR Productions, a Bay Area literary organization, for more than a decade. She also helmed the imprints Sister Spit Books at City Lights Publishers and Amethyst Editions at The Feminist Press. She produces and hosts the Your Magic podcast, wherein she reads tarot cards for Roxane Gay, Alexander Chee, Phoebe Bridgers, and other artists, as well as the live tarot show Ask the Tarot on Spotify Greenroom.